NURSES AND THEIR PATIENTS: COMPASSION AND COMMITMENT

A Short Story Collection

By Lois Gerber, RN, BSN, MPH

ISBN 978-0-9885706-1-0

'Nurses and Their Patients: Compassion and Commitment' is a collection of stories based on the author's experiences as a community health nurse. The primary players are fictionalized composites.

The story, *Tommy, the Angels and Me,* has been taken from 'The Human Side of Nursing', the first book in the series, 'Nursing in the Neighborhoods'.

This book is dedicated to my grandchildren,
Amanda and Owen

TABLE OF CONTENTS

THE SAND DOLLAR

The greater the obstacle, the more glory in overcoming it.

Moliere

Saturday morning and her weekend off, free from work for at least forty-eight hours, Lauren forgot she was a nurse and slipped on a hooded sweatshirt and tugged it down over her hips. She ran a brush through her short light brown hair and headed for the beach. Too chilly for going in the water, but she loved to remove her shoes and walk barefoot in the soft Florida sand.

After standing on her feet for fifty or sixty hours a week in the hospital emergency room, she cherished the moments away from her job. And away from her family. At night she had dreams of being picked apart by grasping hands. Everybody wanted something from her, and she had spent her life giving, giving, giving.

Lauren treasured the two hours on her day off when she walked on the beach. There she saw tourists, happy to be away from the freezing northern climate and locals sitting on colorful terrycloth towels in front of their vans. Children screeched in delight as the ocean water chased them across the sand. Lovers walked along holding hands, oblivious to the world around them. She was glad to be away from the homeless people seeking shelter and comfort in the hospital waiting room or the first-aid they couldn't afford to have treated by a private doctor. For many, by the time they came into the ER on stretchers, it was too late. Lauren cringed when she saw their shriveled bodies.

Homeless people, especially the women, frightened her. She'd grown up in a block of apartments in Daytona Beach that accommodated the underprivileged. Nearly every household, including hers, was familiar with the welfare office. There was hardly enough to eat by the end of the month when the food stamps ran out.

Lauren, the youngest of her family's six children didn't know she was poor until she started school and the kids made fun of her clothes. By the time she received her sisters' hand-me-downs, they were faded, out of style, and stained.

Her mother didn't care. "You're lucky you got clothes, Girl. Don't complain."

When Lauren was in middle school, she started to use the local library to borrow books and find information for school research projects. She read the newspapers there and learned about the world. She realized she didn't have to be one of those welfare people, a bag lady, like the women she saw clustered around the stark wooden tables in the library pretending to read books, when all they were really doing was being comfortable, using the public bathrooms to clean up, and making believe they were normal people. Lauren couldn't stand the smell of them. The urine stench made her want to throw up, so she avoided them. By the time she was eleven, she had developed a pathological fear of becoming a bag lady.

But, in spite of her fear, Lauren couldn't get the homeless women out of her mind. She worried about them and wondered where they went for health care. Where did they sleep?

Her tremendous anxiety about becoming a bag lady drove her to get an education, to find secure employment so that she would never be in that vulnerable position. Lauren worked hard in high school to earn scholarships and even harder in college to keep them. She graduated with honors from the nursing program and went straight from school to work in the hospital's emergency room. She'd been a staff nurse there for fifteen years and eventually had a decent shift, days, seven to three, with every other weekend off.

Lauren was frugal with her money, managing it carefully, making sure there'd be enough for a rainy day. At the same time, she gave an allowance to family members to supplement their meager incomes. She bought a small house for herself but then worried about meeting the monthly mortgage payment.

She dated Mark, a good friend, whom she'd met in her high school geometry class. He felt like a brother; people even said they looked alike with their athletic builds, hazel eyes, and light brown hair. Over the years, he often asked her to marry him, but she never felt the deep love connection she expected. They had great sex; he slept over from time to time; and he even helped her clean up after meals, but she just couldn't bring herself to become his wife. Mark's attitude toward life was too casual for her. He liked to 'live for today, tomorrow be damned!' Good enough for him, because he grew up in a nice house with three bedrooms and a swimming pool in the backyard. He'd never been hungry because his mother ran out of food stamps before the next allotment was due.

* * *

Lauren half jogged across Atlantic Avenue, between the oceanfront houses and down onto the beach. The wind whipped at her hood. She stopped to remove her shoes and socks, tucked them beside a small boulder, and then headed down to walk along the water's edge. After several deep breaths to clear her head, she tucked her hands in her pockets and walked south, skipped along dodging the incoming waves, feeling free for a little while.

She was completely lost in thought, wondering where she and Mark might have dinner tonight, when she bumped into someone.

"Sorry," she said automatically, as she moved to skirt around the person.

"No, my fault, Ma'am." Even with the sea breeze blowing strongly, she smelled the woman before she actually saw her. A homeless woman! A bag lady!

"No problem," Lauren pulled the hood of her sweatshirt more snugly around her face.

"Damned foot!"

Lauren had started to move away from this waste of human life but turned back when she heard that.

"What's wrong?"

"Twisted my damned ankle when you bumped into me. It's nothing."

Lauren started to protest but looked down at the offending foot instead. She cringed at the sight of the filthy knee-high athletic socks and torn high-top sneakers. Her nursing instinct took over. "You'd better sit down. Over here on the dry sand. Let me take a look at it."

"You a doctor?" the woman asked suspiciously.

"A nurse. ER."

Instead of sitting, the woman picked up her right foot and flexed it. "It seems fine now. You don't have to bother."

"Are you sure?" Lauren felt relieved she didn't need to touch this woman's body. With no clean sink, latex gloves, or antiseptic soap handy, she wanted no part of her.

8

"I'm sure. But, could you spare a dollar so I can get some breakfast?"

She smiled at Lauren, exposing crooked yellow teeth.

Lauren took a step back and looked at her. Short, maybe five foot three, salt and pepper hair, but not very old. She'd put her around forty-five or fifty. God, a bag lady wearing olive green shorts and a stained yellow T-shirt under a ragged multi-colored cotton jacket and carrying a backpack slung across her shoulders. The outfit vaguely reminded Lauren of something she'd worn in grade school when the kids made fun of her. She reached into her jean's pocket and pulled out a five-dollar bill. As she handed it to the woman, she looked into her crystal blue eyes and shivered. She felt a peculiar kinship with this odd little person, an idea she wasn't sure she liked.

"Thanks. Thanks a lot, Lady. My name's Stella." She pocketed the money but didn't turn to leave.

Lauren wasn't ready to get on a first name basis with a bag lady. "Yes, well, I've got to run."

"You love the beach as much as me. I can tell. C'mon. What's your hurry? Keep me company for a few minutes while I rest my poor foot." Stella limped gamely over to the sea wall.

Lauren had to smile at the artless ploy. She followed Stella and sat, keeping a good distance between them. She listened as Stella talked.

"Chicago. That's where I'm from. Oldest in the family. Parents alcoholics. I left home two days after graduating high school and never went back. I don't even know what ever happened to my brothers and sisters. Alcoholics, too, I imagine. But, you, you're a nurse. What would you know about being poor and hungry?"

"Trust me. I know what being poor and hungry means." Lauren found herself telling the bag lady her own childhood story of life in poverty. But she felt hers had a happier ending and tried to downplay her accomplishments. "Every day is a worry. Will I have enough money for the mortgage? How much will the insurance rates climb? And, my boyfriend, how long will he wait for me to make up my mind whether to marry him?"

When the sun was high in the sky and the weather warm enough to satisfy the Chamber of Commerce, they parted. Lauren returned to work on Monday and forgot about Stella; but the next week, when she arrived at the beach, there she was waiting for her by the boulder. They walked for a while in companionable silence, then sat down at the same place on the sea wall they had been the previous week. This time Stella talked about her years as a corporate secretary for a financial planner in downtown Chicago. She had earned enough to live in a nice apartment; but after a few years, she became disillusioned about her boss. "He created these pyramid schemes. What he did was technically legal, but he knew and I knew, he was just bilking people out of their money. I complained, and he fired me, said I had an attitude problem."

"That stinks."

"Not working was even worse. Unemployment wasn't enough to pay my apartment rent. My cousin who lived in a suburb west of the city let me move in with her. That didn't last long. She kicked me out after two months."

"What happened?"

"She was an uptight pain in the ass, that's what happened. She didn't like my casual ways."

Lauren interpreted that to mean the cousin thought Stella was a slob.

"Anyways, I went to live in one of those transient hotels in the Loop. You've seen 'em on TV or in the movies? They're worse in real life."

Lauren nodded. "Didn't you look for work?"

"I tried; but, without references, what are you goin' do? My old boss, he was the only person I could use and he didn't like me. I didn't know how to make up a resume, couldn't find a decent job. I guess I could've worked in a fast food joint, but I was better than that. I'd had a good job in an executive's office, lots of responsibility."

"Hmm," Lauren said.

"Anyway, can't change the past. I refused to go on welfare. Not Stella. Too good for handouts. I took to the streets. Carried my stuff in a knapsack and stayed downtown by the water. When it was freezing outside, the police chief let me stay in one of the precinct bathrooms at night."

"Weren't you frightened?"

"I was in a police station! What could happen? In the daytime, I roamed the streets of Old Town. I began singing, yelling, and even talking to strangers. I thought I was being friendly, but people seemed scared of me, pulled away sometimes. Part of me knew I was acting crazy, but I couldn't help it."

"You could've been killed." In spite of her fears, Lauren found that she liked talking to Stella.

"A public health nurse found me one day and took me to a clinic. They gave me pills, called my problem a bi-polar disorder. The medicine evened me out, but I felt flat. Dead. Kind of. No motivation to work or get back into a traditional lifestyle. Life became way too much for me. I went back to my cousin's place and told her about getting on medication, but she only offered to buy me a one-way ticket to Florida. On the bus. And here I am." Stella smiled at Lauren with a crooked grin.

* * *

They spent many Saturday mornings together. Lauren enjoyed listening to Stella, who may have gone unnoticed in a crowd of homeless people if they had they not literally bumped into each other that Saturday on the beach.

Stella explained her life as a homeless bag lady. How she loved to walk the beach, so daytimes were the best. When it was cold, she sneaked into restaurants and hid in the bathrooms. The managers of places who knew her let her stay. More often, she got caught and thrown out. Then there was the library, where the security guards were more lenient.

Stella wore no watch. The sun and the moon were her clocks. "I know when I'm tired, and I know when I'm hungry. That's the only schedule I need."

"But, how do you do it, not having any security in your life?"

"I live for the now. It's all we have, you know. I don't plan for the future. I do things that give me joy and leave me feeling peace. I never did want my life to be only working, eating, cleaning, and sleeping. To be honest, Lauren, I don't know how you do it, all that work and worry."

That last comment startled Lauren. The homeless bag lady thought her life was a drudge. But, when Lauren thought about it, Stella was right. Her work in the ER left her little personal time, and that time was taken up with other responsibilities, like cleaning the house, shopping, caring for her aging parents and shiftless siblings, going out with Mark and doing the things that interested him. Every time they talked, Stella's life seemed more appealing. Lauren marveled how the gulls followed Stella when she fed them bread crumbs. Stella watched for starfish that washed up on shore and threw the live ones back into the water before they died. When she walked on the Main Street pier, a school of dolphins showed up for a visit, knowing Stella would have tidbits of food for them.

She explained to Lauren, "Nature is part of who I am. Who we all are. I feel a special connection to the ocean life."

Lauren felt a sense of oneness with the ocean, too, but she

certainly never displayed it like Stella. Her bag lady friend had no fear or embarrassment about feeding or handling the wildlife. She didn't worry about germs, diseases, or the rising cost of health care.

Stella chatted with other beach goers, tourists as well as locals, homeless or otherwise. She listened intently as if what the others said was the most important and interesting information she'd ever heard. She never offered advice but encouraged the talkers with well-timed touches and personal reflections.

Lauren admired the easy way Stella had with people. Even though she was a nurse and comfortable talking to patients, she felt self-conscious in social situations, preferring the professional less personal ER nurse style of communicating. One day, as she watched Stella relate compassionately and naturally to strangers, Lauren had a thought she considered ridiculous. I've found a mentor in a homeless woman, a bag lady.

"What's your secret for being so easy with people?" she asked her friend.

"I spend hours alone, so when I meet someone, I feel fresh." Stella grinned. "Not everybody likes being around a smelly old woman. That's another reason I like the beach. The breeze dissipates the odor a bit. But, being easy with people? There's no trick to that. I love people. When I'm with them, I focus on them and not on myself. But, I need my solitude, too. That's when I figure out who I am, why I'm here, and where I'm going."

"You make it all sound so simple. I keep trying to scale down my life, but it'll never happen. Too many people tugging me in too many different directions."

"I know. You have your house, probably a car, books, furniture. Things! I have no things. Nothing. I read in the library, so I don't need books or bookshelves. I pick the newspaper from the trash every day, so I'm up to date on who's killing whom."

"I can't believe you're typical of homeless people. You're educated. Philosophical."

Stella laughed out loud. "Lauren, honey, people are people all over the world, and each and every one of us is different and special. Even you! I'll tell you, my time on the beach has put me in touch with a Higher Power. When I worked in the office, my mind was cluttered. My life was cluttered. Can you see me in a high rise apartment with crystal drinking glasses and fine china on the table? Me in a silk peignoir waiting for a boyfriend to show up?"

Lauren had to laugh as she shook her head. "No, actually, I can't."

"That used to be me. But not anymore. Living the way I do now gives me a deep peace. I'm glad I live near the beach and get to meet all different sorts of people."

Lauren frowned as she considered Stella's comments. "But, like you, I think people are basically the same. We all have similar emotions. We might express them differently, but they're the same, nevertheless."

"You're right about that. Everyone wants to feel loved and accepted. Unconditional regard and respect. It's what we're in the world to learn."

"Have you really learned all this from being on the beach?"

"Not really. But being on the beach has helped me change my focus from what's trivial to what's really important."

Lauren gazed out over the waves pounding the shore and the sea gulls flying overhead and had a fleeting thought to try out Stella's unencumbered lifestyle.

Stella, seeming to read her mind, said, "I don't think this homeless thing is for you, Honey. Maybe, spend more time walking on the beach. Not on a schedule, but whenever your spirit needs it. More time on the beach will open your heart, connect your emotions to your mind." Stella reached into her shirt pocket and pulled out a perfect sand dollar. She handed it to Lauren. "Keep it. It will help you to focus on the important things in life."

* * *

The following Saturday, Lauren was disappointed not to find Stella sitting by their rock. She asked around, but no one had seen her. She walked on her own for a while, and then went home, hoping to find her the next day. She even checked the admission list at the hospital, but Stella's name was not on it. When she didn't appear by the boulder the next week, Lauren walked all around town trying to track her down. She looked in the library, the restaurants Stella had mentioned, and the homeless shelters, hoping that Stella had changed her opinion of them.

"She loved being in Daytona. At the beach," Lauren said to a friend of Stella's, another homeless woman.

"That's the way we homeless are, how we live. Here today. Gone tomorrow." She held out her hand, and Lauren dropped a dollar bill into it.

"Let me know if you see her."

"I will, Lady. Stella liked you."

* * *

Lauren never found Stella, but she wore her sand dollar on a brown leather cord tied around her neck to remind her of the homeless bag lady who had once been her friend. She took more interest in her homeless patients now when they came through the ER and searched for the right shelter and other resources for them.

She even started to carry bars of soap on her weekly jaunts to the beach and handed them out to the needy. She became known as the 'Soap Lady.' And when Lauren heard that an abandoned hotel was scheduled for demolition, she organized a network of businessmen and other caring individuals to rescue the building,

15

renovate it, and turn it into a temporary homeless shelter and health care clinic for the poor.

Now, instead of fearing homelessness, Lauren began to dream about being a bag lady on Daytona Beach. She would like to have the sky as her ceiling, the ocean and sand as her floor and walls. She could bask in the sun and listen to the never-ending waves pound against the shore. She could fall asleep under the shimmering moonlight; and when she woke up, the stars would be her nightlight. Her spirit could travel with the wind, fly away high in the sky with the pelicans and sea gulls. But these thoughts remained only a dream, a dream created by the fond memories of Stella, her bag lady friend and mentor.

* * *

The headache began late in the day while she hooked up an overweight middle-aged man to an EKG machine. He'd just been brought in by ambulance suffering with chest pains. Within moments, her head hurt so badly, she had to excuse herself and find someone to relieve her. She headed home, barely able to see as she drove through the streets. She took three strong pain-killers and went to bed, hoping the pain would be gone in the morning. Too much stress. She clutched at the sand dollar, as she fell into a troubled slumber.

The next thing she knew, she was lying on a stretcher in the ER, looking up at bright lights and fuzzy faces.

She squinted.

"A ruptured aneurysm. Good thing he got you here right away," a doctor told her.

"Ooh," Lauren heard her voice say. She was trying to ask who brought her here, but she couldn't speak. She tried to raise her right arm. It wouldn't move. She recognized Mark's face in the crowd surrounding her and tried to tell him she'd had a stroke, but the words wouldn't come out. She could see the anxiety in his eyes and wanted to comfort him, tell him she'd be all right. She

16

longed to tell him that she loved him and was sorry she'd never married him. If he'd still have her, she would. As soon as she got well.

"I've called your family. Your mother and sisters are on the way," he said.

She didn't want anyone, much less her family, seeing her like this. She was the strong one who gave the others emotional and financial support. She was the problem solver with a listening ear, not the person needing help.

Lauren closed her eyes when an aide led her mother and sisters into the room.

"Lauren, sweetie, we're here. We couldn't believe it when Mark called. I thought he was playing a joke on us," her mother said.

"You can't be sick, Lauren," the sister a year older than her said. "We need you. We love you, too."

Lauren wondered what her father would have said if he had still been alive. Probably, "Who's goin' buy my beer, now?"

Her two sisters parked their mother in a chair and then sat beside her to hold her hands. They both cried and moaned about the ungrateful siblings who hadn't bothered to come to the hospital. Lauren thought the ungrateful ones were probably the ones at work, making an effort to take care of themselves. She wished they would all go away.

When she was transferred to the neurological ICU, she managed to get her point across that the only visitor she wanted was Mark.

He remained by her side through her brain surgery and waited until the doctors told him she should recover. It would take a long time, and she would likely never be able to work again. Her speech had already improved. People could understand her even though her words were slurred.

She knew her head had been shaved for the surgery; nevertheless, she was still shocked to see herself in a mirror after the bandages came off. Not once did Mark seem to care how she looked, but she was glad that her hair had started to grow back in.

Lauren was discharged to a nursing home where she received intensive rehab for ten weeks. At first, former class and work mates came to see her on a daily basis. As the months passed, her visitors came less and less often. By the eighth week, only one or two people would occasionally show up. Her brothers checked in with her a few times. Her mother and two sisters stopped by to visit, too, but never became interested or involved in her care. The three of them would arrive, make a big fuss at the nurses' aides to find them soft chairs, and then sit across the room from her and look at her in silence. She felt like a dying cow in a desert with vultures waiting to pick her body clean.

Mark was the only person who had remained faithful to her during the entire crisis. He was there to help her relocate from a nursing home to a beachside group home where she would receive long term help with day-to-day living, assistance with things like grocery shopping, cooking, and cleaning. She still had trouble moving her right side, eating without drooling, and saying certain words. She used a cane when she walked in unfamiliar territory and needed people to watch out for her safety.

Once she was settled in the group home, Lauren began to believe that she might actually get her life back. She was ready to tell Mark she'd marry him; he'd promised to visit later in the day to see her new room in the group home. She considered all the years she had wasted, fearing the unknown, worrying about Mark's casual attitude toward life, when it had been her own attitude that had kept her from living life fully. Now, at age forty-eight, she felt ready to settle down. Many of her friends from school were already having grandchildren! She smiled as she thought about Mark and her walking down the aisle. She picked up the phone and invited him to come for a visit. Her heart skipped a beat when he agreed.

* * *

The day of Mark's visit Lauren dressed in a peasant skirt and short-sleeved white blouse. She asked an aide to help her brush her hair and apply make-up. Then, she sat down to rest in the chair beside her bed to wait for him. Thoughts of their future life together swirled through her head.

Mark walked into her room, carrying a small bouquet of carnations. "Some flowers for you, Lauren."

She smiled. "Mark, sit over here, next to me. I want to talk to you about something."

He set the bouquet on the bureau and sat opposite Lauren. "I wanted to tell you something, too. I have good news."

She looked into his bright brown eyes and could see the happiness in them. Was he so glad to see her recovering? Maybe she wouldn't have to say anything except 'yes.'

"Go ahead, you first," she said.

"I've asked Andrea to marry me," he said proudly.

"Andrea. Who's Andrea?" His words didn't make any sense.

"You don't remember her? I met her the night I brought you to the hospital. She was the nurse on duty. I don't know where you've been hiding her all these years, but we've been seeing each other ever since, and as neither of us is married and we're …" He stopped. "You're upset. I thought you'd be happy for me. I would never do anything to hurt you, Lauren. I love you. I've loved you from the start, but you never wanted to marry me. You said no so many times."

Lauren couldn't stop the tears from falling. "You're right. I'm just being emotional. The move. I'm really happy for you, Mark. I have my life, and I always knew it would end up being me with

19

me. Now, go on and be happy with your Andrea. I'm sure she's a lovely woman, a nurse even."

He squeezed her hand. "I'll still be here if you need me."

* * *

Lauren had worked diligently over the years to protect herself from financial disaster, so when she became permanently disabled, her home was paid off and her income adequate to meet her needs.

Even though she had her own furniture and a few possessions around her, she felt like half a bag lady.

She assigned Mark the job of renting out her house and managing her income. He and Andrea visited her occasionally on a Sunday afternoon. Her mother and sisters came the day before most holidays and brought small trinkets from the *Dollar Store*. Lauren's recovery left her with a limp, a slight slur in her speech, and a troublesome drool. Not a pretty sight, she was sure. But she still walked on the beach wearing her sand dollar on a leather strap around her neck, hoping to see Stella again. Wanting to be able to thank her and tell her about the soap and the hotel she'd turned into a shelter. And how people stopped calling her the 'Soap Lady' and started to call her the 'Hope Lady.'

URBAN PAWS: SUBURBAN LAWS

When patterns are broken, new worlds emerge.

Tuli Kupferberg

"Ethan has Asperger's Syndrome, not autism, Diane," the developmental specialist, Freida Newman, told my husband, Tim, and me. "Asperger's is less severe."

We sat on wooden chairs in front of Freida's large mahogany desk piled high with papers. Shelves filled with textbooks lined a side wall; framed diplomas made a chess board out of the wall behind her.

"Oh, my God." My voice cracked. "I've guessed for months something serious was wrong but hoped he would grow out of it. But, when he turned two, I knew he needed to be tested."

"Likely, he'll never grow out of Asperger's, but his behavior can change. With therapy, he can live a normal life. It's good you recognized it so early." Freida set Ethan's chart aside and looked up to meet my eyes.

I swallowed hard. "The worst is that he won't let me hold him when he's upset." The words caught in my throat.

"That's how it is with Asperger's, not much positive response to people and a general dislike for cuddling. Our job is to teach Ethan how to understand human emotions and how to connect to people, something most of us do naturally."

I grabbed Tim's arm. He pulled me close. My eyes filled with tears. Even though I was a nurse and recognized that Ethan wasn't developing socially and had unusual temper outbursts, I wasn't prepared for the emotional upheaval of hearing the official diagnosis, Asperger's Syndrome, spoken aloud by a professional. Could I handle this? I wasn't sure.

Ethan was a skinny baby, lank and lean, with curly blond hair and a light complexion. He rarely let me hold him and preferred playing alone in his crib with his mobile and music boxes. At eighteen months, I worried because he was still not walking and lacked the normal curiosity of a one year old. I blamed myself, thinking I was a bad mother.

The pediatrician told me, "He's fine, Diane, only a little behind. Kids develop at their own pace. All children are different."

For weeks, I researched the Internet. Tim didn't understand. "He's just a little slow like my brother. You worry too much," he said

By his second birthday, Ethan wouldn't make eye contact with anyone except me. He didn't respond to the overtures of other children and kept apart from people, preferring to be alone. His favorite activities were playing with his number blocks and watching the same Barney DVD over and over. He wasn't even interested in the cake and ice cream at his second birthday party. My biggest worry was his hand flapping, a sign of autism, but I felt encouraged that he'd caught up in language development.

Everything I had read highlighted the importance of early treatment and how it can dramatically improve the lives of many of these children. Only after I hounded the doctor and told him about the hand flapping, did he arrange for the battery of tests by the developmental specialists. The pediatrician's referral ensured that insurance would cover the cost. Yet I'd have followed up anyway, paid for it somehow.

* * *

Frieda was heavily involved in autism research. She alerted us to a clinical trial that used classical music for brain stimulation and auditory processing and referred Ethan to a pre-school program with a special curriculum for children with Asperger's. He was also prescribed a low dosage of Valium, which he took for several months. Tim and I set up a routine that we followed for over two years. I dropped him off at pre-school and then continued my day as a visiting nurse in an inner city health department. Ethan's teacher, Mrs. Hartford, a middle-aged mother of two teenagers had a bubbly personality and related to Ethan and me in a warm easygoing manner. I trusted her competence in developing an individualized educational plan for him.

Ellen Wexford, the petite school nurse with an infectious laugh, gave me practical advice to handle Ethan at home. She suggested making charts and pictures to help plan his day's activities and showed me how to avoid power struggles with Ethan when he acted rigid and stubborn.

"Use concrete examples, not abstract ideas, when you talk to him. Structure every day the same way," she suggested.

When Ethan turned five, Ellen and Mrs. Hartford scheduled a parent meeting to discuss Ethan's progress. Since Tim was working, the three of us sat around a circular table in the school's conference room.

I leaned forward in my chair. "How's Ethan doing?"

Mrs. Hartford tapped her pen on the table. "He's an intelligent kid. He can print all his letters and numbers up to twenty. Just started to write his first name. He only had one temper tantrum this week when we took him away from his number blocks because it was time to eat lunch. You know how hard it is for him to change from one activity to another."

"Number blocks have always given Ethan comfort," I said. "Sometimes, he counts from one to ten over and over, hates to be interrupted. It drives me crazy."

"He still flaps his hands when anyone approaches him, but it's getting better," Mrs. Hartford said.

I took a deep breath. "I have good news. Remember how his grandma used to be scared he would cry when he saw her eyes, so she wore sunglasses around him."

Ellen laughed. "Yes, I remember how hard it was for you to convince her to take them off and let him to have eye contact."

"Last week Grandma made eye contact with him for the first time, the only person besides his dad and me. She was really happy, even cried a little."

"That's a major milestone." Ellen reached across the table and squeezed my hand.

I smiled. "Any better eye contact here at school?"

"A little," Mrs. Hartford said. "We still look him directly in the eye and exaggerate our emotional expressions. Sometimes, we penetrate that steel wall he has and he laughs, and other times, we can't, and he cries and looks away."

"I still feel uncomfortable around my friends. Ethan doesn't interact or talk to them. He often wants to play alone. But, now when there's a group of kids around, he plays closer to them than he used to."

"Have you ever thought of getting a dog?" Ellen asked. "Ethan' relates well to a black lab, Toby, that Dr. Newman brings in for her research study on pet therapy for autistic kids."

I was eager to hear her thoughts. "How so?"

"Ethan pats Toby, gently too. Granted, a little hand flapping is still there, but the kids often do that when they're excited in a happy way. And he looks Toby in the eye. I've watched him very carefully."

Not sure that getting a dog was an idea I wanted to commit to, I said, "Tim and I will have to talk about this," all the while thinking, no way. They're too much extra work. I was already living a thirty-six hour day. Ethan's therapies, doctor's appointments, my job. Most nights I fell asleep in my chair watching the evening news. Yet if it would help Ethan….

* * *

Already behind on my home visit schedule, I drove away from the suburban pre-school in a reflective mood, thinking how much I had wanted a dog as a kid and begging my parents for one. I remembered my mother's fear of dogs.

"They can bite when they don't get their way," she'd warned me.

"Too messy for a house," Dad had said.

But this is different and if it would help Ethan….

* * *

The dogs in the inner city neighborhood where I worked lived in doghouses and stayed outdoors most days. Families depended on them to guard their homes. They barked and snarled at anyone walking by. But would a dog help Ethan? I wasn't sure. I mulled the idea over in my mind as I drove from one client's home to the next. Maybe a dog, but definitely not an inner-city mutt. A pedigreed would be a safer choice.

My last nursing visit that day was to a middle-aged woman, Mrs. Kallenbach, who lived in a small ramshackle bungalow with a dilapidated green doghouse in one corner of the family's muddy postage-stamp back yard. A tan and white collie mix lay close to the fence. When I neared the home's cyclone gate, the dog jumped up and furiously barked. Her husband came out of the garage and put the dog on a leash. I scurried through the yard onto the front porch.

"Don't worry. She's protecting her puppies. There are three of them, just seven weeks old, in the cardboard box there next to the doghouse door," Mrs. Kallenbach told me as she welcomed me into the home.

Once we were inside, we went into the patient's bedroom. I washed my hands while the patient lay down on her bed so that I could take her vital signs and check the infected wound on her ankle.

"I'm glad you're here today, Diane," Mrs. Kallenbach said, while I changed the bandage covering the wound. "You wouldn't happen to want a puppy, would you, Honey? They're a yellow lab/border collie cross mix. My husband's going to drop them off at the pound tomorrow, can't find anyone around here to take 'em."

I thought what an unusual coincidence this was. "I'll take a look at them."

Mrs. Kallenbach smiled. We headed out to the yard to check out the puppies. I was surprised how excited I felt. Should I take one home for Ethan? They were all so cute. Which one should I choose? When I picked up the dogs, the only male, a mop of beige and white fur, snuggled up under my chin. Suddenly I changed my mind about getting a pet, and a *Heinz 57* variety to boot.

"Could you hold this one 'til late tomorrow afternoon?" I asked Mrs. Kallenbach. "It's for my son, Ethan. He has lots of trouble relating to people."

"I guess, Honey. Just for you. We'll wait 'til four o'clock to drop them off. The puppy you're holding is the friendliest of them all, very alert and playful."

"I've never had a dog before. Are they a lot of work?"

"Honey, they're a piece of cake. Feed 'em and put 'em outside to poop and run around a little. That's it. City dogs are different from those fancy suburban dogs. City dogs take care of themselves. They don't need special coddling, can think on their feet," Mrs. Kallenbach said. "It's in their genes."

How ridiculous. No way. Everyone knows animals operate on instincts, whether they live in the city, suburbs, or a farm.

I hugged the puppy before leaving the Kallenbach's. Already I was thinking of how to introduce him to Ethan and Tim. Even though my husband had grown up on a farm with many animals, he never wanted a pet.

He often said, "Dogs need to live in an open environment. I hate the way people baby their animals today."

To prepare Tim for the idea, I parked my car and called him on my smart phone.

"What? Get a dog. We never talked about this," Tim shouted into my ear. I pulled the smart phone back. He often reacted negatively to a new idea initially, only to change his mind later.

"Ellen Wexford thinks a dog would be good for Ethan. She tells me how he connects to the black lab at the school."

"Hmm, I'm not sure. He won't help take care of it. We'll have to do that."

"A dog might be less threatening to him than people. You know how direct eye contact terrifies him. Mrs. Wexford says Ethan looks the school dog right in the eye and smiles."

"What kind of dog are we talking about?"

"He's the cutest thing, tan and white, fluffy, a border collie/lab mix."

Tim softened. He'd do anything for Ethan. "Okay, we'll try it for a month, see how it works out." he said. "For now, I need to pick up Ethan. It's five o'clock. We won't tell him 'til tomorrow,

27

maybe after breakfast, until we talk about this some more."

"Thanks, Love. I'll take care of dinner tonight." I disconnected from my smart phone and eased the car back on the road.

Later that night after Ethan rocked himself to sleep on the side of his bed, I heard pounding from the basement. I crept down the cellar steps to find Tim tacking down a piece of blue carpet to an old bureau drawer that had been sitting in the garage for months. "For the dog," he mumbled.

"It's beautiful." I walked over to hug him. Sheepishly, he kissed my cheek.

The bed was not quite what I had in mind. I'd planned to buy a tan wicker basket with a plush red cushion. Keep your mouth shut, I told myself. He's already bought into the dog. Don't ruin it.

I knew tomorrow we'd get the puppy and that he'd be here to stay.

* * *

The next morning while we helped Ethan dress for school, Tim and talked to him about Toby, the dog at school.

"Do you like him?" I asked our son, as I brushed the tangles from his curly brown hair.

He waved his arms back and forth. "I like Toby. He's nice."

"Mommy and Daddy want to get a dog, a little puppy just for you."

Ethan jumped up and down. "Yes, my very own dog. When?" He looked directly into my eyes and laughed. Then, he ran over to his toy box, pulled out a stuffed Dalmatian, and said, "I'm going to name him Spotty."

* * *

After work that afternoon, I drove to the Kallenbach's to pick up the dog. Quickly thanking them, I carried the puppy to my car and put it in a cardboard box with a threadbare beige blanket for the ride home. Tim and Ethan were waiting for me.

"Spotty, Spotty, Spotty," Ethan exclaimed, as he picked him up. When the dog nuzzled up against his shoulder, he laughed.

I smiled. The puppy had found a new home. And now he had a name, too.

Spotty lived inside our house but loved the outdoors. That summer he learned to let himself outside by pawing open the lock on the screen door. He practiced jumping the chain link fence until he could scale it. A few times, I had to track him down, as he ran in circles through the subdivision yards.

One day, when Ethan and the dog were chasing each other throughout the house, I took them both outside to quiet them. The strategy worked. While Ethan sat on the porch stacking his numbered blocks one on top of the other, Spotty guarded him, sitting proudly a few feet away and taking this new responsibility seriously. He barked loudly when anyone approached, alerting me to any possible danger. It was the only time Spotty accepted being tied up outside. What a relief to find such an easy way to keep them both occupied.

Ethan was a fussy eater. Spotty ate everything in sight. Ethan giggled when he dropped food on the floor and Spotty gobbled it up. Soon Ethan put his plate on the floor, sat down and ate most of his meal from his lower vantage point, Spotty at his side. Both he and Spotty loved marshmallows for dessert. After two weeks of sitting on the floor to eat, Ethan returned to the table, a better mannered diner for all our efforts.

One Saturday afternoon, Tim and I heard the front screen door slam. Various thoughts circled my mind as I looked out the window. Looking at Tim, I said, "I can't believe that dog is out again. I had left the door tightly locked with a little piece of masking tape over the latch."

He bit his lip. "Let's wait a bit before I go look for him."

Ten minutes later, I spied Spotty with a huge brown boxer by his side, jauntily walking down the sidewalk.

"That's Roman," Tim told me. "New to the neighborhood. I talked with his owner last night, nice guy about our age."

I nodded. "Look who's with them. Ethan. He was playing in the sandbox a minute ago. He must have just run out from the back yard."

"Let's follow them. They look like they're on a mission," Tim suggested.

The threesome stopped to check out a tennis ball lying on the sidewalk. Ethan picked it up. Out ran another boy, who looked to be a year or two older than Ethan. "That your dog?" the boy asked. "Roman's mine."

Ethan pointed to Spotty. "He's mine."

"You're lucky. He's cuter than Roman. What's his name?"

"Spotty."

"You wanna play?" the boy asked.

Over the weeks, as Roman and Spotty became buddies, Ethan and Sean became friends. Sean had a younger brother with cerebral palsy; probably that's where he'd learned the patience to deal with Ethan. The two boys and the two dogs often played together, mostly throwing and catching tennis balls. I was ecstatic. Ethan was actually relating. The next week, Mrs. Hart- ford told me he was playing interactively with children at school, too.

Many Saturdays and Sundays, Sean came knocking at our back door with Roman scratching the screen with his paw, a signal for Spotty and Ethan to 'Come out and play'. Ethan laughed, grabbed several tennis balls from the hall closet, and ran out the door with Spotty. I don't know who had more fun—Ethan and Sean who threw the bright yellow balls or the dogs who fetched them.

* * *

At Ethan's year end conference, I sat on a wooden chair in front of Mrs. Hartford's desk. She smiled. "Keep up what you're doing at home with Ethan. It's working."

I breathed a sigh of relief. "It's partly the dog. Spotty helped him connect to a boy in the neighborhood. And the school had a big impact, too, of course."

Mrs. Hartford picked up the pencil on her desk. "Until last month he spent most of his time playing by himself with blocks and building things, maybe some Hot Wheels cars. Now he's talking me to the other kids; he even plays creatively with the Star Wars figures."

I swallowed hard. "He's almost a normal six-year-old kid."

My heart did flip-flops when she said, "We'd like to schedule him to begin kindergarten in a regular classroom next year."

* * *

That summer, we took a family vacation, the first time Ethan had been calm enough for us to travel. The car was full—Tim and me in the front seat and Ethan, Spotty, and Grandma in the back. The windows were opened to let in the cool breeze. We stopped at an intersection in a small rural Ohio town where men and women were relaxing on their front farmhouse porches. In a split second, Spotty jumped out the window to chase a calico cat and ran right onto the cat owner's steps. Tim pulled the car off the road, and Ethan and I jumped out.

"You've got a feisty one there," the farmer laughed as we went to retrieve the dog.

"I'm so sorry," I mumbled. "Damn dog."

"Thank you, Mister. Spotty's a good dog, not a damn dog," Ethan said.

* * *

Occasionally, I allowed Ethan and Sean to bring the dogs in the house to play in our unfinished basement. The two boys went through three boxes of *Milk Bones* and a bag of *Oreo* cookies teaching the dogs to sit, shake hands, and stand on their hind legs. Sometimes, neighborhood kids stopped by to join in the fun. On Halloween, the boys tied *Darth Vader* bandanas around the dogs' necks and took them trick or treating to the immediate neighbors.

Although still shy in his kindergarten class, Ethan made one new friend, Ashley. Once for 'Show and Tell', he brought in a photo of Spotty and Roman and told the kids stories about the antics of the two dogs. When he received B's and C's on his report card and did especially well in math, I was happy. The school year passed quickly.

* * *

"What's wrong with Spotty?" Ethan asked one day. "He doesn't run good anymore when he plays ball."

Ethan was right. The veterinarian. Dr. Hart, diagnosed a brain tumor. Over the next few months, Spotty's condition steadily worsened. When he could no longer walk, Tim and I knew the end was near. Dr. Hart suggested euthanasia.

After dinner that evening, the three of us sat around the kitchen table. The opened window let in a soft breeze. Tim looked at Ethan and covered his small hand with his calloused one. "We have some sad news about Spotty," he said.

"Oh no. I know what you're going to say. Spotty's going to die, like Sean's parakeet. He found him lying on the bottom of his cage one morning. He couldn't move anymore. " Ethan's voice cracked and tears came to his eyes. He jumped up from the table and ran into the den.

I went to him and held him close. "You're right; his body is going to die. His legs aren't working, his head probably hurts him; he's very sick like Sean's parakeet was. He'll always be our special dog. We'll have him for a few more days, enough time to say goodbye." I swallowed hard.

He cried into my shoulder. When his sobbing stopped, he pulled away and looked at me. "I want another dog, just like Spotty," he said.

I nodded. "We'll see what Dad thinks."

He wiped his face with the back of his hand. "Okay. I'm going over to Sean's house now."

* * *

Later that night, Tim and I had just turned out the lights and had gotten into bed. "It was hard telling Ethan about Spotty," I told him.

"I know," he said, "but how wonderful that he can mourn a loss, feel the emotional pain of loving and losing. He wouldn't have cried last year."

I hugged Tim. "Ethan really is getting better. Hard to believe the change."

"We're all doing better, Diane," he said.

I squeezed his arm. "He wants another dog."

Tim smiled. "Of course, we'll get another dog."

* * *

Several days later, Grandma babysat Ethan while Tim and I took Spotty to the veterinarian to be euthanized. Dr. Hart lifted Spotty onto the treatment table. "You made the right decision to bring him in. He's not happy anymore living the way he is. He's been a tough dog, one of my favorites."

Tim and I stood on the other side of the treatment table. As I stroked Spotty's shaggy fur, he turned his head to the side. Tears formed in my eyes as Dr. Hart injected the medication into his vein. Seconds later his heartbeat stopped and he lay still.

* * *

Goodbye, Spotty. Maybe it was Frieda Newman, Ellen Wexford, or the therapy, or the special school, or Sean, or the

Johnsons or Tim and I that helped Ethan get better. Then again maybe it was you that allowed Ethan to heal, make the transition from relating to things to relating to people. You lived in the suburbs but never became a suburban dog. You kept your urban personality to the end.

THE HOCKEY PLAYERS

Sports do not build character. They reveal it.

Heywood Broun

The puck slid across the ice and into the net. I stood up and cheered. Two to two. My Detroit Red Wings were putting up a good fight against the Chicago Black Hawks, our big rival. When the Black Hawk coach called a time-out, I sat down and relaxed.

The falling snow brushed against the window that January night. The wind whistled through the trees, making the house seem as drafty as an outdoor ice arena.

I wanted to be at the Joe Louis Arena to see the game in person. Instead I sat on the sofa beside my pregnant wife, Larissa, watching the hockey game on ESPN. By now I had given up my dream of becoming a professional player; the seven college hockey trophies on the windowsill were as good as it was going to get for me. Three years ago I graduated from Northern Michigan University with my finance degree, married Larissa, and started to work for an investment firm in a Detroit suburb.

When the players returned to the ice and the Red Wings took

control of the puck, I leaned forward.

Larissa touched my arm. "The game's not that important, Kevin. Put your hand here. You can feel the baby kick."

My voice choked as I gently touched her swollen belly. "He's alive in there, and he's moving. Soon, I'll be a dad."

We knew our first baby would be a boy, my son, perfect, and a hockey player just like me.

Just before the final bell, Larissa grabbed her stomach and shrieked, "Oh my God. I'm wet. My water broke! The baby!" My wife clutched the sofa pillows, her eyes wide with fear and anticipation.

I snapped the television off. My son, eager to be in this world, would be seven weeks premature. He would live. I would see to it.

I jumped up and called her obstetrician, Dr. McGuire. "There's blood on Larissa's slacks."

"Bring her right in. I'm at the hospital," he told me. After wrapping Larissa in a blanket, I carried her to the SUV and carefully placed her on the back seat. I ran my fingers through her dark brown hair and kissed her on the cheek. Then I closed the rear door and slid into the driver's seat.

Her voice cracked with fear. "Hurry, Kevin, please."

The back wheels of the van slipped as we inched up a hill. Even with the defroster on high, a thin coat of ice formed on the windshield. I straightened my shoulders and leaned forward to look through the small circle of clear glass. The rhythmic swish of the windshield wipers and my heart pounding in my ears were the only constants in my little world. In spite of the danger, I kept my foot on the gas pedal and ran through a red light. Tires screeched. A horn honked.

"Kevin, it hurts. Hurry!" Larissa cried.

"I'm doing my best, Honey. Just another couple minutes." Beads of sweat dripped from my forehead.

"Oh God!" she mumbled. Her words sounded like a prayer.

"Hold on, Sweetheart. We're pulling into the hospital entrance now."

Seconds later, two orderlies opened the car door, lifted Larissa onto a stretcher and wheeled her away. I walked alongside them trying to brush the snowflakes from her hair. I could only mutter, "I'll be right there," before they whisked her through the doors of the hospital's birthing center.

When I entered minutes later, a clerk cleared her throat and pointed to a desk. "You'll need to stop here to fill out the paperwork."

The lines on the form blurred as I scribbled the insurance card numbers in the small spaces. I hoped the clerk wouldn't make me do it over.

Just as I finished, Dr. McGuire approached. "Larissa's in early labor. The ultrasound shows the cord's around the baby's neck and will choke him if we attempt a vaginal delivery. We need to do a C-Section."

"Please don't let Larissa or the baby die." Suddenly, I didn't care if my son played hockey or not. I only wanted him to live.

Dr. McGuire cleared his throat. "Larissa's strong. She should be all right. You'll be a father soon." He shook my hand and walked back into the birthing center.

I found a seat in the waiting room. A sport's announcer was recounting the end of the hockey game I had missed, the game the Red Wings eventually won. Unable to concentrate on the television, I sat with my head in my hands, hoping for the best.

An hour later, Dr. McGuire returned, a smile on his face. "We finished the C-Section. Larissa did well. You have a son. He weighs three pounds, nine ounces."

My voice cracked. "Thank you, Doctor. He's so tiny. Is he okay?"

"Yes, he's breathing a little erratically, but that's normal for his low birth weight. He'll stay in the hospital for a while." Dr. McGuire put his hand on my shoulder.

"But he'll eat, gain weight and be normal. Right?" I jingled the car keys in my pocket.

"We hope so…."

"Does he have all his fingers and toes?"

"Yes, ten of each. But his lungs aren't well developed. We need to watch his breathing."

I gulped. "When can I see them?" "Soon. The nurse will come get you."

* * *

We named our son Andrew. He had light brown fuzz on his head and a red scrawny body. Several times a day, I walked Larissa down the hospital corridor to visit him in the preemie nursery. We either sat beside his special bed or carefully held him between the wires and tubes connected to his little body. One set of wires was hooked to an apnea monitor. The nurses explained how the monitor alerted the staff if his breathing slowed. When I saw him kick, I knew he would be a hockey player after all.

"He'll fill out, won't he? He won't always be skinny and frail?" I asked Larissa.

"He's beautiful just like he is." She had a faraway look in her eyes.

"I know, but…" I stammered. "I want him to be normal. Like other kids."

"Kevin, he'll be himself. Take each day at a time."

Feeling less sure, I clenched my fists and looked out the window.

* * *

Three days later, Larissa was discharged from the hospital, but Andrew had to stay. The neonatal doctor was still concerned about his breathing. "We want to be sure his lungs stay clear," he said.

Larissa's face was pale and her big blue eyes wet with tears as I helped her get into the car. As we drove home, Larissa stared out the window in a daze. "We'll be going to the hospital every day to bring my breast milk. The nurses put it in a bottle with a soft nipple. He's sucking better every day."

"I'm taking time off work to drive you. And I want to feed Andrew, too." I also planned to exercise his little legs every day to make them strong.

* * *

Even though Andrew's breathing pattern remained uneven, Larissa begged the doctor to let us bring him home. I hesitated, afraid we couldn't take care of him properly.

"We'll send a nurse to teach you what to do," the neonatologist said.

Three weeks later, we brought Andrew home, strapped in an infant car seat with his apnea monitor beeping quietly next to him.

Annette, the visiting nurse, came later that day. She taught us more about the apnea monitor, how to stimulate Andrew when his breathing slowed, and how to perform CPR if that didn't work. She listened to his lung sounds, and carefully monitored his weight and overall development.

* * *

Over the next several weeks, we watched our son gain weight and grow. He sat on his own at eight months and was crawling by ten months. I relaxed. Andrew seemed normal after all.

Right before his third birthday, he developed a cold and a wheezy cough. The pediatrician ordered a ten-day course of antibiotics. Two months later, he became sick again. "I'd like to check him periodically. It could be an early sign of asthma," the doctor said.

"Will he be all right?"

"I think so. We'll watch him carefully."

I looked the doctor in the eyes and vowed to myself to make Andrew tough, so he could play hockey just like me. "I want him to be like other kids."

* * *

When Andrew was four, we had another baby, Shelly, a girl this time.

Our third child, another daughter, Suzanne, was born a year later. Both pregnancies were normal.

Andrew became his mother's little helper. Larissa was content for him to be indoors. I wanted him to be outside kicking a ball or playing with his trucks in the dirt.

When Andrew was almost five, he began to cough after running or crying hard, and several months later, he developed a significant wheeze.

We took him to an allergist.

"The asthma is mild, activity induced. I'll prescribe an inhaler. Have him take one puff if he wheezes or has problems breathing after activity," the doctor told us.

Larissa watched our son carefully, letting him play outside for fifteen minutes at a time. She made him wear a knit cap when the temperature dropped below sixty-five degrees.

"Quit babying him," I said. "He needs to play outdoors for as long as he wants, develop his lungs for hockey."

Larissa was firm. "He's better inside. He's just a child and a kid who picks up colds easily."

I let Larissa have her way. Andrew rarely needed his inhaler any longer, and he seemed to be outgrowing his asthma. Time would be on my side.

* * *

By the time Andrew entered second grade, he was a short skinny boy with blond hair, blue eyes, and a ready smile. When his younger sisters and their friends asked him to play house or dance to *Barbie* DVDs, he obliged. I hated to see him play girl stuff; it's not what I wanted for my son.

By third grade, his nose always seemed to be in a book. He read and re-read the *Harry Potter* series. I introduced him to the *Jack London* wilderness stories-boy stuff. At bedtime every night, I read to him from the biography of Bobby Orr, the greatest hockey player in the world.

"I like it when you read to me, Dad," he said as he snuggled into my shoulder.

* * *

For his ninth birthday, Andrew begged for CDs of Itzhak Perlman.

"Who in the heck is Itzhak Perlman?" I asked.

"Only the greatest violinist in the world."

I scratched my head. "So?"

"I want to play the violin when I get to middle school," he told me.

I mentally rolled my eyes and agreed, thinking he'd change his mind when the time came.

* * *

The winter he turned ten, Andrew announced, "I can't wait to take violin lessons. Alicia in my class takes them at the conservatory. I want to, too." He handed me a flyer that showed the sign-up was three weeks away.

I brushed the flyer off the table. "How 'bout hockey?"

"Aw, Dad, I don't like skating. When you and I go out on the ice, I get cold. I fall down a lot. I don't skate good like you."

"Every time you play, you'll get better. I started to play hockey when I was eight. I wasn't that good back then either."

"I wanna learn to play the violin, take lessons."

"This is a good year for you to start hockey. I have a surprise. I'm going to be an assistant coach for the Pee Wee hockey team this year."

Andrew looked down at his feet and kicked the floor with the toe of his sneaker. "Okay, I guess hockey could be fun, just you and me. How 'bout if I take violin lessons and play hockey, too?"

I thought for a minute. "Okay, Son, it's a deal."

* * *

Later that evening Larissa came into the den where I was watching ESPN. She sat down next to me on the sofa. "Don't force him to play hockey. He's not a sports person like you."

I looked up from the television. "He'll be a man someday. He needs to do boy stuff like hockey. All he does is play around the house with his sisters and their friends. I don't want him a 'pretty boy'."

"Kevin, you're being manipulative," she said in her slow serious voice.

I moved closer to her. "He wants to play the violin. What if we let him do both? We'll rent him a violin for six months and see how he does. You can find him a teacher."

The look in her eyes told me she would agree. "All right. I don't like that he plays with the girls and not boys his own age, either. You do your hockey thing. And I'll hunt up some violin lessons. But be careful. His asthma. Don't let him overdo."

"Don't forget, I love him, too; I only want to toughen him up. Since I'll be part of the coaching squad, I can keep an eye on him."

Larissa took a deep breath and nodded.

* * *

At the after-school hockey orientation in the ice arena's locker room, Andrew and the other *Pee Wees* stood in line waiting to get their hockey jerseys. When the coach handed Andrew his shirt, he slipped it on over his sweater. He was the shortest boy on the team, and his jersey hung almost to his knees. I smiled thinking how his size would be to his advantage if he learned to skate fast and shoot the puck accurately.

I took his hand. "Let's drive over to the *Sports Authority* and get your skates and the rest of your equipment."

He looked down at his shoes. "Having a special shirt is the best part. I like my number. Eleven!. I don't want to buy skates or play hockey. I'm scared I'll fall down a lot."

"You'll be fine." I said as we walked to the arena's parking lot. Once we were settled in the SUV, I flipped on the ball game. Andrew sat in the passenger seat staring out the window.

It was a short drive to the *Sports Authority*. The minute we walked into the store, Andrew walked over to the rack of professional hockey jerseys. "You pick out what I need while I check out these hockey jackets."

"No. Get over here. You need to help me choose the right stuff and try on your skates and helmet."

He sauntered over and tried on skates and a helmet until we found some that fit. I selected the rest of his equipment for him.

When we got home, Andrew carried the purchases to his

bedroom and lined his helmet, shin pads, and hockey stick up in a row in the back of his closet. I felt encouraged.

* * *

Practices were twice a week and at six-thirty in the morning. It was hard to wake him up early enough to get to practice on time; some days he had to eat his breakfast cereal in the car.

In the middle of the season, Larissa and I lingered over dinner sipping a second cup of coffee. "It's too much for him," Larissa said. "He's looking tired. You shouldn't push him."

"Let me be a father." I picked up a newspaper article about parenting and handed it to her. "Read this. It says fathers need to teach their children self-reliance and how to function in the world, something dads do better than moms."

She pushed the paper aside. "Kevin, you need to work with Andrew's interests, not force him to be like you. You should read some parenting books."

I stomped out of the kitchen. Andrew stopped me on my way to the den. "I heard you two arguing. I like being with you, Dad, but I hate hockey."

I felt my face turn red. "Give it one season. If you don't like it then, you can quit."

He looked down at the floor and jammed his hands in his jean's pockets. "All right."

* * *

As part of the coaching team, I made sure Andrew started every game. His tongue inched from the corner of his mouth just before he swung his stick. His legs wobbled when he skated and his timing was off, so he missed a lot of shots. Two other fathers complained that I played him too much, but I didn't care.

I set up a practice area in our basement to teach him defensive moves. At first, I had to bribe him with a chocolate sundae from

Dairy Queen to work with me. He urged me to slow down and not to hit the puck so hard, which forced me to ease up a bit. Eventually, his game improved, and he became a decent but not outstanding player. The shortest boy on the team had grown taller than me; he was still skinny but had firm muscles in his arms and legs.

Since he played in every game and the team won several championships, I thought he liked hockey. After strenuous skating sessions, his breathing became labored, but two puffs of the inhaler quickly resolved the problem. I was happy he was participating and didn't see it as a problem.

Larissa and his sisters cheered us from the stands right through his middle school years. The tiny black jersey became a small green one, then a medium blue one, and then a large red one. Several wooden trophies with engraved brass plates sat on his dresser next to the framed photos of him and his teammates. His were much nicer than my tarnished and warped ones still sitting on the den windowsill.

The night after we won our district championship, I was in the den watching a basketball game on television. Andrew sauntered in and said, "I'm quitting hockey and joining the Junior Thespians. Acting fits in better with my violin. Hockey practices take up too much time."

A shiver shot through my chest. I had so many more plays I wanted to teach him.

"Dad, I'm done. Don't make me play anymore. I want to join the drama club and act in the high school play. My English teacher agrees. So does my music teacher."

He stomped off to his bedroom and slammed the door.

I went to the kitchen to find Larissa standing at the counter drinking coffee.

"Dammit, Larissa," I yelled, "Andrew's not going to be some

sissy actor, all dainty and girly. My son's going to be a real man."

Larissa handed me a cup of coffee. "You have to let him be his own person. Maybe he's not cut out for hockey. Yesterday, he told me that he'd worked himself up to the first violin chair in the high school orchestra. You only saw one concert. The girls and I rarely miss his performances."

I shrugged. "I felt he was being covered. And I was busy with hockey. I can't do it all."

She shook her head. "You know you could have done more."

I poured some *Baileys* into my coffee and took a sip. "What if he's gay? Remember my Uncle Sterling? My friends used to make fun of him, the way he swished when he walked and how he wore his hair in a pompadour. Called him a queer. I don't want that for Andrew."

"He's not gay; maybe a little different. He told me the other day he had been playing hockey to please you all these years. He never really liked it. He wanted the two of you to be together and make sure you loved him."

I gulped. "He never told me that."

"He was afraid of you, Kevin. He's going to join the acting group. I told him, 'Go for it'. It's what he wants. He's not you."

"What if he's gay?"

"You will love him anyway."

I put my hands to my face and rubbed my forehead. "Dammit, I don't know if I can, Larissa. I feel bad, but I won't push him to play hockey anymore."

She squeezed my hand. "I'm glad."

* * *

Andrew had the lead in the spring play, *Peter Pan*. He gave us all tickets in the center section of the third row. I didn't want to go

46

and see my son act like a girl.

The next day, Larissa and I were planting flower seeds along the front walk. "You must go to the play, Kevin," she said in a firm voice, more firm than I had heard for years.

I was taken aback and set my trowel down. "Why? It's not that important."

She squeezed a clump of dirt. "He needs your support. It's only one night, a couple hours."

I looked at her angry eyes and felt the disdain in them. "Just this once, Larissa. I don't support his acting idea."

Andrew played the *Peter Pan* role well. He received a standing ovation. I stood up but didn't clap. I felt embarrassed the character was so feminine.

* * *

In his senior year of high school, Andrew announced that he planned to spend his spring break in the Florida Panhandle. The three of us were sitting in the den watching a DVD. "Everyone is going, the drama club kids, even my old hockey friends."

I clicked off the remote. "It'll be a free-for-all down there. I don't want you part of it. There's alcohol and drugs. We don't want you to get hurt. You're too young and too easily influenced to handle it." My voice was firm. "No compromise".

Larissa agreed. "I worry about your asthma, Andrew. You're not thinking this through."

He pounded his fist of the table. "My breathing has been fine for months. Stop treating me like a baby. Alan's driving us all in his dad's van. I'm going whether you let me or not. I've saved enough money."

"You won't be able to handle it," I said.

"I can handle it. I'm seventeen!" he hollered. "It isn't fair." He stormed into his bedroom and slammed the door behind him.

47

I looked at Larissa. "He's not strong enough. He'll follow the crowd."

"He's rugged on the inside, Kevin. He's had to be to live with you. And he's never been one to follow the crowd."

I nodded and took a deep breath. "I guess you're right."

I leaned back in my chair and wondered how this angry young man, the little preemie that I once held so gingerly in my hand, became the way he was. By now I was reconciled to the fact that Andrew would never play hockey, but this disrespect. Why?

Larissa put her hands on her hips. "He is almost eighteen. Kevin, I've watched you put him down for years. Enough is enough. He's a good kid. I say we okay the trip. You've always wanted him to be a man."

I stomped outside to the back yard and picked an empty bird's nest from an evergreen and threw it on the ground. Why can't children be as easy to parent as baby birds? Knowing Larissa would have her way, I felt angry yet afraid for Andrew at the same time.

* * *

The day the boys left on their trip, my stomach lurched as the car full of teenagers pulled out of our driveway. I walked back into the house, sat down on the recliner in the den, and flipped on ESPN to a Black Hawks and Red Wings game. Listlessly watching the Red Wings score, I thought of Andrew and hoped he was all right.

His asthma had improved a lot in the last couple of years but....

* * *

Sunday, the day the boys were scheduled to return home, I was watching another hockey game on television. A weather alert flashed on the screen. "A late spring ice storm has hit Ohio. Interstate 75 from Dayton to the Michigan border is treacherous."

Oh, my God. No bad weather here, but that's about where the boys would be. "Larissa, there's a storm. I hope they're okay." I took a deep breath.

She came into the room and squeezed my hand. "You have to have faith, Kevin."

Ten minutes later the phone rang. "Mr. Keller, this is Officer Mullins with the Ohio State Police." I pushed the remote button to flip off the television.

My voice quivered. "It's about my son, Andrew, isn't it? What happened?"

"There was an accident, a fender-bender. No one was hurt. We arrested Andrew. He was driving with a false ID and his blood alcohol level was .15. We're holding him in the Toledo jail. He insisted his friends drive the van home. He didn't want to cause them trouble."

"Oh my God. Andrew's in jail? "

"We're a little worried. He's slightly short of breath and mentioned he has mild asthma. He said he lost his inhaler while traveling. Is there a way we can get him the medicine? He says he's fine but we don't want to take any chances. The roads are bad here. We'll plan to keep him overnight."

"Thank you, Officer. But I'll come down and get him. I'll leave here soon."

I ran my hands over my face. Tears came to my eyes. Why did we let him go? Drinking and driving. How could he do that? Stupid kid.

I clenched my fists. "God dammit, Larissa. If it wasn't for his asthma, I'd let him sit in jail overnight. The storm's headed our way. Listen to the wind."

"I'll come with you. We'll need to take his inhaler. There's one in the bathroom, in the medicine cabinet. I'll get it." She came back with the inhaler in her hand, then went to over to the closet and pulled out her coat. Tears ran down her cheeks.

I wiped them away and held her close. "No, you stay here with the girls. I'm sorry. I'm upset. We can't leave him there," I whispered.

Larissa pulled back and brushed her fingers across my forehead. "Call me when you get there."

She handed me the inhaler and I stuffed it in my pocket. My thoughts went back to the night Andrew was born and how I drove Larissa to the hospital in that terrible snowstorm. What if I lose him now? I couldn't bear it.

* * *

After entering the police station's address into my GPS, I pulled my SUV out of the driveway and was on my way. The roads were still dry in Detroit, but the sky looked cloudy, perhaps an omen of the storm predicted to begin soon.

Once I crossed the border into Ohio, the roads turned to a sheet of ice. My SUV slid. I nearly crashed into the center median but recovered just avoiding a head-on collision. I began to sweat even though the air in the car was cold. The windshield wipers left streaks of ice on the glass. I drove at a slow steady pace and pulled behind a salt truck. When I saw the highway exit to the police station, I gave a silent prayer of thanks.

* * *

The officer brought Andrew to me from his holding cell. He ambled into the waiting area, his hair disheveled, his eyes glassy, yellow stains on the front of his white T-shirt. I was prepared to engulf him in a long bear hug, but I stopped short. This derelict couldn't be my son. A ball of fire took over my gut, and bile rose to my mouth.

"I can't believe what I'm seeing. I was so worried about you. Now I'm pissed off. Making me drive to get you in this weather.

50

What you've put me through all these years."

"Dad, thanks for coming. I'm sorry for…everything, not being the son you wanted." He coughed and began to breathe fast. I pulled the inhaler from my pocket and tossed it to him. He must have been sober by now, because he caught it midair and took two puffs. The officer led us to a small scratched wooden table. We sat across from each other on metal folding chairs.

Andrew was breathing normally now. He looked at me with pain and hurt in his eyes. "I want to get out of here." He covered his face with his hands.

I grabbed his shoulder. "Come on. The officer said I could take you home."

"Dad, the roads are bad. We should stay overnight in a motel here in town and go back tomorrow."

"Don't be a wuss. Straighten up. Go to the men's room and comb your hair. We're headed home. I'll show you how a man drives. A little snow doesn't freak him out."

I felt my face grow hot and could taste bitter acid on my tongue. How could I have raised such a wimp? It was all Larissa's fault.

* * *

After I signed the papers, we left the police station. Feeling the blood pumping through the veins in my neck, I walked ahead of Andrew and got to the car first. He was ten steps behind me, struggling to keep up.

Andrew closed his eyes and swallowed hard when he got in the car and slammed the car door shut. He folded his arms in front of him and refused to look at me. He turned his face toward the passenger window, but I caught him wiping a tear from his sunburned cheeks. I knew I'd made him feel bad, and I was glad. Once I inched the car onto I-75, the traffic was almost at a stalemate, inching along in the right lane where two ruts of ice had formed. Snow swirled across the windshield blurring my vision for seconds at a time. I could feel my heart pound in my chest like a drummer in college football bowl's half-time shows. My hands were white where they clenched the steering wheel. I gave the car in front of me the finger and mouthed, "Get out of the way."

Andrew gaped at me. "Dad, no!"

I pulled myself up closer to the windshield. "The snow and ice isn't that bad. I can drive in all kinds of weather. Snow, sleet, ice, driving rain. Just watch your old man."

I steered the car out to the left and put my foot on the gas pedal. A horn honked, then another. Brakes screeched. I lost control of the car and shrieked, "God dammit." My world turned black. I woke up covered in snow in a ditch on the side of the road. I tried to move my arm but couldn't. When I turned my head to the side, the snow was red with my blood. I thought of Larissa in labor and the blood on her clothes when I drove her to the hospital. My leg, my back, and my neck throbbed. I couldn't stand the pain.

Andrew stared down at me. I felt my son's fingers firmly hold my arm. "Dad ...."

Two police walked over to us. One of the officers spoke. "It was a bad accident. Three other people were injured. Your son here's okay. He saved your life, stopped the bleeding with pressure."

"I need something for pain. My back's killing me."

"I'm sorry," the officer said. "We called the EMT. They're on their way, but it's slow. Until then you'll just have to grit your teeth, be a man."

The ambulance transported me to a Toledo hospital. Andrew sat beside me, anger still in his eyes. When the emergency room doctor said I needed surgery, my heart pounded. What if I die! I looked at my son, dirty T-shirt and all. Overnight Andrew had turned into a man, someone I wanted close by.

I swallowed hard and looked deep into his eyes. "I'm sorry I've pushed you to be someone you're not. I see now you're a man, a good one, thanks to your mom. Please stay with me. Don't let anything bad happen."

My son gave me a sheepish grin and squeezed my hand. "I'll be here, Dad. You know, I've never seen you like this. I like you better when you're not so tough."

"In case I don't live through this, I want you to know I love you, always have."

He looked at me with a new softness in his eyes. "Somewhere in here, I always knew that." He laid his hand over his heart. "I just called Mom. She's driving down with the girls when the snow stops. Kendra asked about you too."

"Kendra?"

"Yeah, a girl in the Thespians with me. She's real nice. I think you'll like her."

"A girl?" My whole body relaxed, like a slab of concrete was lifted from my shoulders. Not gay then. Good. But right then I realized it didn't matter. He was my son and he was a man.

A QUESTION FOR MR. DAVE

We do not remember days, we remember moments.

Cesare Pavese

Melissa looked up at Dave, the school nurse. "I love you, Mr. Dave. Can I hug you?"

He gently pushed her aside, keeping a hand on her shoulder, as he did with many of his Down Syndrome students. "I like you a lot, Melissa, but I can't hug you. Remember, you must not rub your body against mine or any of the teachers."

Melissa sulked back to the examining table. She was in the nurse's clinic at a special school for teens with Down Syndrome. This was Melissa's third year there. She had just turned sixteen.

Earlier in the afternoon, Melissa had complained to her teacher that she had a stomachache, so she could get out of class and go to the clinic to see Mr. Dave, who had gray eyes and blond hair styled like Jesse McCartney's. She loved to look at the photo on his name tag and read the words, David Andrews, RN, under it. Once she had tried to unpin the name tag when he was busy writing in his charts so she could take it home and keep it under her pillow. But Mr. Dave pulled away and told her not to touch it.

Melissa liked it when Mr. Dave listened to her heart beating and the gurgling sounds in her stomach. Sometimes, he put the stethoscope in her ears so she could listen, too. And every six months, he weighed her on the big scale and measured how much she had grown with a yardstick glued to the wall. Most of the time, Mr. Dave was fun.

Not today. Today Mr. Dave acted tired like her daddy did when he came home late from work. "Where does your stomach hurt?" he asked, pointing to different places on her body. Melissa giggled.

"Are you sure you have a stomachache?" he said.

She laughed again. "I wanted to see you and talk to you. I love you. Uh, oh. I just remembered that you told me not to say 'I love you'." Melissa chuckled.

Mr. Dave finally smiled. "You're right. I'm glad you remembered."

"Can I be your girlfriend?"

"What would my wife say? And my kids? Remember I'm your nurse, not your boyfriend."

Melissa pouted. "No one loves me."

"You know how your mother and dad take care of you. That's love."

"What's boyfriend love?"

"That's a special kind of caring. It's about wanting to be with this one special person, a boy, and liking him a lot. It may happen when you are older, Melissa."

Melissa frowned and then laughed again. "Maybe I'll find a real boyfriend someday, just like you, Mr. Dave."

He patted her arm. "But for now, Melissa, go back to class."

* * *

The following year, because Melissa's seventy IQ categorized her as a high functioning Down's student, she was mainstreamed into a public high school. Melissa felt confused at her new school even though she was assigned a personal assistant who accompanied her to most of her classes and tutored her on any material she did not understand.

Melissa wished she were back in her old school.

"Give it a month," her mother told her. "It's good you can go to the regular school. You'll learn more there."

"I feel lonely. No one likes me."

"Say hello to the other kids. Hang around with your friends from the old school, the group that transferred with you."

"Yesterday a boy called me a retard. 'You're a retard too', I told him, but he just laughed." Melissa started to cry.

Melissa's mother hugged her daughter. "Some kids, and some grown-ups, too, don't know how to be kind. That means not saying anything to hurt someone else's feelings or make them feel sad or afraid."

"I'm kind."

"You are, and I'm very proud of you."

"I'm trying really hard to be smart like the other kids."

"In some ways, you're smarter than the other kids. Maybe not with books and numbers, but with liking people and getting along with them."

"I want them to like me."

"Some of them will, and some of them won't. It's like that with all of us. You're very brave, honey. It will work out. Just wait and see."

"Okay. I'm going to watch *Sesame Street* now." Melissa's mother tousled her daughter's light brown hair. "Good idea," she said. The following week Melissa still felt sad. She seldom went to the football games, and didn't understand why the other kids got so excited about the Friday night festivities. She didn't join any of the other extra-curricular activities and never went to the school dances.

* * *

She was excited when her older sister asked her to be a bridesmaid in her upcoming wedding. She liked her sister's sparkly engagement ring. "Can I try it on?" she begged.

"Just for a little bit, Melissa. You have to give it back when *Dora, the Explorer,* is over."

"Okay." Melissa said, getting up from her chair in front of the television. First she put the ring on her index finger, then she took it off and held it up to the sunlight coming through the window. It's beautiful, like a twinkling star."

She started to sing 'Twinkle Twinkle Little Star.'

After Melissa returned the ring to her sister, she told her mother, "I want a boyfriend too."

"Someday maybe. We'll see," her mother said, as she cleared the dirty dishes off the table after dinner.

"What's 'boyfriend love' mean anyway?"

"Love for boyfriends is hard to explain, Melissa. It's about feeling good when you're around one special boy and doing nice things for him. He takes care of you, and you take care of him. It's not easy to find, but it's worth more than anything else in the world."

"It'll be easy for me to find 'boyfriend love' but not today. Today, I feel sad."

* * *

Melissa's mother picked up a yellow sheet of paper from the kitchen counter. "You know, honey. I found this flyer at the library about the Special Olympics' track team. What do you think?"

"Maybe. I like to run."

"The team will train for three months before the big race." "That's a long time to practice."

"Yeah, practice is twice a week right after school on the outdoor track behind the YMCA."

"Can I go swimming there, too?"

Her mother smiled. "Not right now, Melissa. Maybe this summer."

"All right, I'll try the running, then."

* * *

Melissa liked training for the Special Olympics on the track at the Y. She was excited when she met Jimmy, an eighteen-year old boy also born with Down Syndrome. Jimmy was a high school graduate who lived in a group home and did piece work in a sheltered workshop program.

Melissa liked looking at his blue eyes and shiny wire-rimmed glasses. She wished she had a pair of glasses like that. Her frames were brown plastic. She tried to stay close to Jimmy so she could run beside him.

"I can run faster than you," Melissa challenged him one day before they started practice.

"No, you can't," he hollered as he took off down the track. When he tripped over a tree root and fell, Melissa was scared. She ran over to him and wiped the dirt off his face with the sleeve of her sweater. He was already standing when the coach approached.

"Are you okay, Jimmy?" the coach asked.

Jimmy straightened his glasses. "I'm all right," he said.

"I'm sorry you fell," Melissa told him.

"It's okay," Jimmy answered as he patted her shoulder.

The friendship flourished. Melissa couldn't wait until Tuesdays and Thursdays, practice days. She wore her special jeans and had her mom style her hair with the curling iron. Sometimes, Melissa and Jimmy took a break from running and sat on the grass talking about everyday things: how to make peanut butter and jelly sandwiches, the pretty weeds around the track, and how to give Jimmy's dog a bath. When the coach passed by, he didn't say anything. He just looked at them and smiled.

One day the team went to *Baskin and Robbins* for ice cream after the practice. Melissa and Jimmy sat beside each other. Tentatively, Jimmy stroked Melissa's hand, then squeezed it and gently held it. "You feel sweet. I like you," he said.

Melissa felt proud that Jimmy said the 'like' word. She remembered how Mr. Dave had taught her not to say 'I love you' to anyone except family and close friends.

"Want a bite of my ice cream?" she asked.

"Yeah." Jimmy laughed. When he started to lick her cone and got ice cream on his nose, they both giggled so hard Melissa thought she might wet her pants.

They stopped laughing when the coach came over to hand Jimmy a napkin.

"Wipe your nose, Jimmy," he said.

"Want to go to the Homecoming Dance with me?" Melissa asked Jimmy a few days later after practice.

"I don't know how to dance," he said.

"My sister's teaching me. She'll teach you too. Get your mom to drive you to my house on Sunday evening."

"I'll ask her. I like music."

"I love you, Jimmy," Melissa whispered. Then she put her hand to her mouth, remembering what Mr. Dave had told her. "I'm sorry. I'm not supposed to say the 'love' word to anyone but family and close friends."

When Jimmy said, "We feel like family," Melissa laughed and hugged him. She wished Mr. Dave were around to ask how love really felt, what it really meant to be in love. Was love that warm feeling in her stomach?

* * *

The Special Olympics race was the following Saturday. Right before the event, Jimmy told her, "One of us will win. You and me are the fastest runners."

When the starting bell sounded, Melissa got a good start and was ahead of Jimmy by a few feet. She slowed down on a curve and looked back to watch Jimmy run. When she saw the smile on his face and the determined look in his eyes, she realized Jimmy wanted to win the race more than she did. Her parents shouted for her to keep running fast, but she kept her slower pace to allow him get ahead of her and cross the finish line to win the event. She came in second.

The judge pinned a red ribbon on her T-shirt and a gold one on Jimmy's. When he looked at her and winked, Melissa smiled, because she knew Mr. Dave would tell her it was all right for her to say "I love you" to Jimmy now.

TOMMY, THE ANGELS, AND ME

The butterfly counts not months but moments,
and has time enough.   Rabindranath Tagore

The day I turned eight, Mama forgot to make my birthday cake. Grandma had to buy one from the store. When Mama, Daddy, and Grandma sang 'Happy Birthday' to me, and I blew out the candles, everyone pretended to be having fun.

See, my little brother, Tommy, was very sick. He couldn't walk or play with me, and Mama and I had to feed him mushy food with a special spoon and give him a bath in bed. He couldn't even sit up to blow out three little candles when it was his birthday last week. I had to do it for him.

When I asked Mama what was wrong with Tommy, she said. "We don't know, Jennifer. Only the angels understand."

Once I heard Aunt Peggy whisper to Uncle Al, "Tommy will never be right." Well, how could Tommy be wrong? He hardly ever even talked.

I hated Tuesdays, the day Dr. McCready came to examine Tommy. The doctor always wore a black suit and looked mean. I didn't like him. He made my stomach hurt. Daddy usually was in a bad mood the day the doctor visited and yelled at me to stay out of the way and not make any noise, not even talking sounds.

Maybe I made Tommy sick when I pinched his leg last Christmas. Maybe that was why he couldn't walk or play with me. I wished I had another brother or sister to talk with about leg pinching. I was too scared to ask Mama or Daddy.

Once when I heard Dr. McCready's car pull into the driveway, I ran into the woods behind my yard and climbed high up into the long branches of a big weeping willow tree. I hid there for a long time chewing on my little finger, hoping Mama and Daddy would be worried and come outside to look for me. They didn't though, and I finally went back to the house. Mama was standing by the kitchen sink with her back toward me looking out the window. Even though I slammed the screen door, she didn't hear me come in, so I tiptoed upstairs.

Soon, Dr. McCready started to visit more often, because Tommy got sicker. The sparkle in his eyes had disappeared. He grew thinner and stopped eating or drinking much, even when Mama tried to give him water through a glass straw, but sometimes he licked sugar from the end of a spoon Daddy slipped between his lips. Unless Mama or Daddy carried him, he stayed in bed usually lying on his back.

In the summer, there was no school, so I played outside a lot to stay out of everyone's way. My friends, Nicky and Susan, told me I wasn't fun to play with anymore. Most every afternoon, I hid in my special tree.

One day, a lady in a navy blue suit, a nurse whose name was Ms. Harper, came to see my brother. She visited Tommy every few days and acted different than Dr. McCready. She smiled and talked to me and let me be in the room with her when she took care of Tommy. She showed me how to wash his face with a small white washcloth. I loved to rinse out the cloth and feel the water in the pan slosh around.

She carried a big black purse with a lot of stuff in it. At first I didn't like her things, but after she explained to me what they were, I found them interesting. "This is a stethoscope," she said. "Do you want to try it?"

"Yeah, I guess."

She pulled back my hair and put the ear pieces in my ears. At first they felt funny, but then I got to listen to my heartbeat. I liked to hear the thump, thump, thump in my chest.

Some days Ms. Harper brought me crayons to draw pictures. I drew a big one of Tommy and a little one of me. She asked, "Why did you make yourself small when you're the big sister?"

"Cause he feels bigger."

She sighed. "Hmm. Sounds like you feel small sometimes."

I looked down to the floor.

She knelt beside me and gently lifted my chin so that we were at eye level. "You're very important. Mama, Daddy, and Tommy need you a lot. You help them smile, just by being you."

I thought about this. "Maybe." I picked up my ball on the floor and bounced it.

Ms. Harper patted my head. "They're lucky they have you around."

One morning when I got up, Tommy wasn't in his bedroom. I hunted for Mama and found her in the living room. "Where's Tommy?" I asked.

"Sit down, Jennifer." she said. My heart started to beat fast.

Mama looked me right in the eyes and whispered, "Tommy's with the angels now. He's very happy. We won't see him for a long time." She stopped talking for a few minutes. I figured she wanted me to say something, but I didn't know what. I looked down at my feet.

"Why would he go away?"

She said, "It's for the best. The angels wanted him."

"Why can't I have him?"

"The doctor couldn't make him better."

"How come?"

"Sometimes questions don't have answers. I wish they did. I have to go out with Daddy now. Grandma's in the kitchen, and she'll stay with you."

Mama wouldn't look at me, and I knew she wouldn't say anything else and that I shouldn't ask any more questions. She glanced out the window, grabbed her gray purse off the coffee table, and walked out the door to get in the car with Daddy.

I ran back to the bedroom to make sure Tommy wasn't hiding under the blankets. I couldn't find him anywhere. I rushed out to the front porch and sat on the top step and waited for him to come home. For the whole rest of the summer, I sat on the same step every day after lunch and watched for Tommy to walk up the street. I thought maybe the angel would come with him and tell me why he was sick for so long and why he went away.

* * *

One afternoon in September, when I was sitting on the steps, Ms. Harper drove up the driveway. The minute she stepped out of the car, I noticed her crooked smile and almost laughed.

She put her arm around my shoulder. "Hi, Jennifer, You look pretty today. Maybe the two of us can talk after I see your mom."

"Okay." I opened the door for her to go inside.

When she came out, I was still sitting there.

"Jennifer, what are you doing on the steps? Are you waiting for someone?" she asked.

"I'm waiting for Tommy," I replied. "Mama said he went to heaven with the angels but that we'll see him someday."

She sat down beside me. "Oh, Jennifer, I can see you're sad. You miss your brother, and that's okay. Tommy can't come back to see you."

"How come?"

"His body won't let him."

I started to cry. "Why?"

"He died. His body stopped working, just like those brown leaves that fall from your special tree."

"But where is he now?"

"Now he lives is in your heart."

I tapped my chest. "How can he be in here?"

"Because you can remember him anytime you want. When you think of him, you'll see his face inside your head."

I tested her idea. I thought of him, and he appeared in my mind. He was smiling, and his eyes were sparkly. "I can see him!" I told her.

"You can always see him that way. But you can't see him with your eyes anymore like you could when he was alive, but he'll always be with you."

"I get scared, Ms. Harper. Mama and Daddy get upset when I ask them questions about Tommy."

"Mama and Daddy don't answer your questions because they are so sad they can't talk about him. They miss him too."

"They're mad at me. They think I made him get sick."

Ms. Harper hugged me tight, and when she pulled back I saw a tear in the corner of her eye. "No, Honey, you didn't do anything to make Tommy sick. No one knows why Tommy had a bad growth in his brain. It made his body slowly stop working, and then he died."

"No, I did it. I made him sick. When I pinched him, he cried, and Daddy said I hurt him. He yelled at me." I stood up and kicked the back of the steps. When I rubbed my eyes, Ms. Harper handed me a tissue. I bunched it up threw it on the ground.

"Lots of kids get pinched, you know. They don't get sick."

"No, but Tommy got sick right after that."

Ms. Harper put her hands on my cheeks and turned my face toward her. She looked at me with her dark brown eyes. "I promise you, Jennifer, that the pinching had nothing to do with Tommy getting sick."

"I wish I didn't pinch him."

"Lots of big sisters pinch little brothers sometimes. Tommy forgot about it quickly. He knew you were sorry."

"I shouldn't have pinched him though. Daddy said he was special. Why was he the special one and not me?"

"Daddy and Mama think you're very special."

"Then, why did he get to eat sugar right from the spoon and sleep in Mama and Daddy's room at night?"

"Mama and Daddy knew his head hurt, and they wanted to make him feel better. They would have done the same for you if you were sick."

"Why did he go away, somewhere he can never come back from?"

"I don't know, sweetheart. Maybe his life here was finished.

The part of him that you remember will always live. The important person now is you."

"No, nobody likes me anymore."

"We'll talk more about how you can be happier. I'll visit again and bring you a present."

"What will you bring?" I smiled.

"Maybe some tulip bulbs to plant in the woods by your special tree. When we first put the bulbs in the dirt, you won't see anything growing. Next spring though, green leaves will peek through the ground and after that, beautiful flowers."

"What color will they be?"

"All different colors. Just like both you and Tommy have many different parts to who you are. Think of Tommy's life as a tulip—a beautiful brother who couldn't be with you very long. When he died, he started to live in a new way, a way that's hard for you to understand. Sometimes there's life in hidden places. The tulip bulbs are alive under the ground even though you can't see them now. Tommy's alive now in a way that you can't see."

"Will I get sick like Tommy?"

"You're strong and healthy and very special. Your body's not like Tommy's"

"Will I die, too?"

"Someday we will all die like Tommy, and people will miss us too like you miss Tommy. I think your body will live for a long time."

* * *

When I turned nine, Tommy wasn't there to watch me blow out my candles. Now I understood that Tommy would never come back to play with me, and I stopped sitting on the steps. Months later the tulips that Ms. Harper and I planted sprouted. One April afternoon, I saw three green leaves. Soon there were bright red, pink, and yellow flowers. I watered them almost every day until the petals died and fell off the plant. I called them 'Tommy's Tulips.' That's when I started to play with my friends, Nicky and Susan, again.

For a while I thought the angels had forgotten me. I never saw anyone floating around with white robes or heard voices from the sky. But maybe some angels live on earth and are nurses, wear regular clothes, and talk like normal people. Maybe Ms. Harper was one of those angels.

When I get big, maybe I can be an angel, too. Or, even better, maybe I will learn to become a nurse like Ms. Harper.

THE HOMECOMING

Sometimes the heart sees what is invisible to the eye.
H. Jackson Brown, Jr.

I heard the screams, "Nurse Aly, Nurse Aly," before I opened the door of my rental car. It was Kim! After eight years of being away from Alaska, I could still recognize her voice.

She stood in front of the Fairbank's walk-in clinic where I used to work. I looked at the grown-up Kim, probably twenty-two years old now, and saw a trim and fit young woman with long black shoulder length hair. She wore tight white slacks and a long sleeved black sweater, very fitting for this cool summer day. The young girl with poker-straight black hair and dark brown eyes standing beside her must be her daughter. A splitting image of her mother. I smiled, happy that Kim recognized me after all these years.

* * *

Kim had been one of my favorite patients. I first met her ten years ago. Her aunt, a short buxom woman about thirty years old, brought her to our clinic late one morning. Back then Kim was a skinny young girl with long thick hair who wore a navy parka and heavy woolen pants.

"She's got the nits," the aunt said. "She don't live with me. Her ma and pa are working in the lumber yard today."

70

I smiled as I generally did when first meeting a new family. Head lice, a nuisance problem easily spread from person to person, is often hard to get rid of in this primitive rural area. "I'll be glad to check her out. For starters, hang your coats up on the hooks over there. Then, we'll sit at the table here and you can tell me your names and addresses, that kind of stuff."

Fifteen minutes later, I'd been introduced to Anna Birdsong and her twelve-year old niece, Kim. Once we had finished the paperwork to open her case, I said to Anna, "Let's go into one of the examining rooms, and I'll take a look at her. "

I put on my latex gloves before separating the strands of Kim's thick hair. I was shocked to see the lice, mounds of them the size of quarters, not nits like her aunt said. "You have a lot more than nits here," I told Anna.

"Fix 'er then, nurse," she said. "Kim ain't a talker but she minds good."

Clearing up Kim's head took a lot of fixing. Anna was right. The girl was quiet and compliant. She even agreed to have her hair cut to a short shag. Over an hour later, after I had removed the black undulating mounds of lice, I found much of her scalp to be infected. I shampooed her head and then applied a creme rinse, *Nix*, prescribed an antibiotic pill to resolve the infection, and sent her home with enough *Nix* to treat all immediate contacts. I instructed the aunt to wash all the bedding and towels the family had recently used. Lice were a common problem, one I was used to treating, but this was the worst case I'd ever seen. The way Kim stood with her right shoulder lower that her left one bothered me. On examining her closer, I noted her left hip was higher than her right one. Scoliosis, likely mild and easily treated with observation and maybe a brace. I sent her across the hall to see Doc Raines, knowing he could order the X-rays needed to make a definite diagnosis.

After X-Rays and an MRI confirmed that the problem was

scoliosis, Kim was fitted for an upper body brace that she needed to wear twenty-three hours a day. At first she was resistant. "I can't wear this thing. It's too stiff," she said. "All my friends will make fun of me."

"It's how you handle it," I told her. "Show the kids your brace, tell them why you need it, and act positive about it."

Perhaps Kim followed my advice, because no one made fun of her. After she showed her classmates the brace and explained how it would keep her from having surgery, the kids autographed it with *Magic Markers*.

Sleeping on her back was difficult for a few nights, but she adjusted quickly as children often do. Every six weeks, Doc Raines and I observed her spine for changes. After several months, the curvature had lessened.

* * *

A year later, as I was getting ready for bed, Anna Birdsong called our emergency hot line. "Nurse, my brother, Jimmy, Kim's dad. He was hit in the head. There was a lot of blood but it's stopped now. He's drunk but a happy drunk."

"Where is he now?" I asked.

"Lying on sofa. I put a towel under his head. Can you come? I'm scared. I've never seen this much blood before."

"Is there any way you can bring him to the clinic? I could meet you there."

"No Ma'am, no way."

Since I needed a partner to make a home visit, I called Todd, an American Indian nurse who worked in the clinic with me. His voice sounded groggy when he answered the phone.

"Did I catch you sleeping?" I asked.

"Uh huh. I was tired and went to bed early."

I cleared my throat. "We have to make a home visit. Jimmy Birdsong, head laceration. Lives out by the state park. We'll call the doc if we can't steri-strip it."

"Quite a drive with the snow and all. I'll pick you up in a half hour."

* * *

Anna welcomed us into her small stucco home. She pointed to a back bedroom, mouthed 'Kim' and whispered "She's afraid to come out."

Just as Anna had told me on the phone, Jimmy lay sprawled on the sofa, his head tilted back. He snored softly. After Todd and I took off our stocking caps and parkas and hung them on the back of a kitchen chair, we washed our hands. I shook Jimmy's shoulder.

He inched open his eyes. "Hhhey. Whaaat you want?"

No doubt that he was drunk, the bloodshot eyes, the alcohol breath, the slurred speech. "We're the nurses from the clinic," I said. "I'm Alison; this is Todd. We came to look at your head."

He shook his head as if to clear his mind. "I got knocked out at the *Coyote Bar.* Asshole smashed a beer bottle on my head." He reached up and touched the top of his scalp. "Oww. God dammit." When he pulled away his hand, his fingers were smudged with blood.

His shoulder length long black matted hair looked so much like Kim's. Todd and I slipped on latex gloves and used one of Anna's fresh bath towels and our surgical sponges to clean the dried blood and debris from his hair. While we worked, Todd kept Jimmy quiet by telling him stories of hunting trips with his dad and uncle.

"I'm going to need to clip your hair around the cut," I told Jimmy.

After snipping an eighth inch of hair on each side of his wound, I looked at Todd. "This is deep. He needs stitches, not steri-strips."

Todd nodded. "Doc Raines will be furious to be phoned so late. He glanced at his watch. "It's after midnight."

A crazy thought popped into my mind when I touched his strands of thick hair. I looked at Todd and Anna. "We could try something new," I said. "Use strands of his hair to close the wound, tie it together. The cut's not long, an inch and a half or so, and his hair is course."

"Sounds like a medicine man idea," Anna said.

By now Jimmy had sobered up. "I like the idea. No stitches. I hate needles."

That's how Todd and I closed the wound. With Jimmy's lying down and his head elevated on a pillow, we approximated the wound edges, took a strand of hair from each side of it, and knotted them together.

When we had finished, Jimmy smiled at us. "You two are good as Doc Raines. Better than Doc Raines."

I squeezed his shoulder. "You stay on the sofa tonight and sleep. Don't get up. We'll be back tomorrow."

Anna grinned. "I'll watch him," she said.

"Good," I said. "Let me check in on Kim while we're here."

We walked to the back bedroom. The window was opened. The girl was gone. Anna frowned and rubbed her forehead. "Her mother was hiding back here with her. They must have taken off. Jimmy didn't tell you right. Kim's mother was the one who cracked his head opened. After he punched her in the stomach. This has been goin' on for years. Liza finally had enough."

I sighed. "We could have helped her sooner had we known."

Anna frowned. "She didn't want no one to know."

"Where's she going?"

"She'll find her way to Seattle to her sister's. Liza left him once before but came back. She seemed more serious tonight. I'm glad Kim's with her. They'll help each other."

I looked at Todd. "Let's find them before they get too far. Make sure they're safe."

Todd and I put our parkas back on, borrowed two flashlights from Anna, and walked around the immediate area. Then, we got into his SUV and scanned the more distant areas but found no sign of them.

After forty minutes, I was cold and tired. "We should take these flashlights back to Anna and quit looking," I said.

Todd agreed. "I hate these dark winter days. Seven hours of daylight isn't enough. It drives people crazy."

A month later, Anna phoned me at the clinic. "I called to tell you Kim and Liza are okay. They're in Seattle with Liza's sister. Just like I told you."

* * *

Three years later I was at my desk finishing the day's paperwork when Kim, now sixteen, appeared in my doorway Her gaze was shy and uncertain. Her bulging abdomen, swollen ankles, and pale complexion signaled she'd had some tough years. My eyes went to her back; she must have worn the brace as it was ordered as the signs of scoliosis had vanished. I walked over to hug her. "Kim, welcome home," I said.

She laid her head on my shoulder and then pulled back and looked up. "I shouldn't have left Fairbanks back then but I was furious at my dad." She rubbed her hand over her belly. "And now the baby. It's not kicking as much. I'm scared."

"Let's sit down and talk," I said, pointing to two chairs wooden chairs in front of my desk. "Who's with you? Your mom?"

Kim sat in the chair closest to the door. "No one's with me. I begged my mom to buy me a plane ticket back home and she finally did. Aunt Anna picked me up at the airport. I got here yesterday."

I rubbed my forehead. "Where were you all this time?"

"Seattle, mostly. Portland for a while. I begged Mom to come back to Fairbanks with me, but her boyfriend wouldn't let her." She clenched her fists. "Even though I left Fairbanks with her when she smashed that bottle over Dad's head, she wouldn't come with me. My boyfriend, Ryan, wouldn't come with me either. Says it's not his kid, but it is, Nurse Aly. I'm not lying." She blinked hard and looked away. "I'm so tired."

I squeezed her hand. "I believe you, Kim. You've had some rough times. But you're in the right place now. You're home! Lots of people here care about you."

* * *

Two days later, she and I were in Doc Raines examining room. Only this time it was for a problem more serious than lice and mild scoliosis.

Kim squeezed my hand while the doctor examined her; this was her first pre-natal check-up. "I wish I never had sex with Ryan."

"Life's about living and learning. This isn't the time to be hard on yourself." I ran my other hand over her forehead.

Doc Raines examined her gently. "Everything's all right, Kim," he said. "It looks as if you're seven months pregnant. We'll order a sonogram to be sure."

The sonogram showed that the baby appeared to be a girl, healthy except for being small for her gestational age.

Kim smiled when she heard the news. "I'm naming the baby

after you, Nurse Aly. I want her to grow up strong and kind, like you are."

I swallowed hard. "That's the nicest compliment I've had for a long time, Kim. "I'll help you all I can."

* * *

Her Aunt Anna took Kim into her home and became the mother the teenager now needed and wanted. With healthy foods, pre-natal vitamins, and a comfortable place to sleep, the girl regained her physical and emotional stamina.

One month later, with a midwife's help, Kim delivered a healthy but scrawny five pound baby girl. True to her word, she named the baby, Alison Anna Birdsong. In the weeks that followed, Kim learned how to nurture and care for her daughter from the experienced neighborhood mothers and the parenting classes Todd and I now taught at the center. Anna reported that Kim was welcome to live with her as long as she liked. "That niece of mine has turned out okay. She's a good little mother."

For the first year, Kim brought Baby Aly, as she was now called, every month to the clinic for well-baby checks. The infant sat alone when she was six months old and was walking by her first birthday. Kim started back to school to prepare for her GED exam. I couldn't have asked for anything more.

* * *

The week after the baby's first birthday, my brother phoned me that our mother, who lived in Phoenix, had had a stroke. The next day I took a plane back to be with her. Because her rehab became long and complicated, I gave up my Alaska job and moved back to my childhood home in Arizona to care for her. That was eight years ago.

* * *

When I received an invitation to Todd's retirement party last month, I decided to go back to Alaska for a visit. I'd left Fairbanks quickly eight years ago and was only able to say goodbye to a few of my patients. Maybe no one but Todd would remember me, but I wanted to see the beautiful Alaskan wilderness and my Fairbank's friends again.

As I stepped from my rental car, heard "Nurse Aly," and saw the crowd of people welcoming me, I felt as if I never had left. Behind Kim stood Anna and Jimmy and many other people whose faces looked familiar. I choked back tears.

Kim ran up to hug me; her daughter followed two steps behind. "Nurse Aly," Kim exclaimed. "When I heard you were coming, I couldn't wait to tell you my news. I've been accepted at the University of Alaska Anchorage in the nursing program. When I graduate, I want to work in the clinic, just like you used to."

THE NEEDLE STICK

Life is the art of drawing sufficient conclusion from insufficient premises.

Samuel Butler

Carrie felt the sharp stick of the dirty needle, but it took a second for it to register that she'd just stuck herself with a needle contaminated with HIV.

She stared at the blood seeping through the puncture of her latex glove. Her heart pounded. Perspiration dripped from every pore of her body. She raced from the clinic's exam room in a panic and bumped straight into her co-worker, Danielle.

"Dani! I stuck myself!" she cried as she stripped the glove from her hand to show her colleague the bleeding wound.

"Calm down, Carrie," Dani said. "It's not the first time it's happened to a nurse, and it won't be the last. It can be serious, so let's take a look." Danielle tried to soothe her with war stories from her own thirty-year career as a community health nurse, but Carrie was in no mood to be comforted.

"You don't understand. Ms. Krieger is HIV positive! I could have AIDS! I could die!" She collapsed onto an examining table as Dani brought her a basin with warm water and anti-bacterial soap. She sat up to wash her finger. "Oh, God. How could I have been so stupid? I'm always super careful. I've been disposing needles for two years, Dani, and never once made a mistake like this."

"Needle sticks can happen to anyone. Try to calm down. You're not doing yourself any good. And stop squeezing your finger."

"I never thought it would be me. I'll need to get my blood drawn."

"Yep, and you'll have to fill out an incident report."

"I came to work in a bad mood. Brian and I were fighting again last night. I got home late from the immunization clinic, and he was already in bed. I tried to be quiet but woke him up brushing my teeth. He started in on me again about getting a hospital job at the new medical center."

Danielle nodded. "A whole different kind of nursing."

"Brian will never understand working in a hospital isn't for me. I can't tell him about the needle stick. He hates me working here at the health department. He calls our patients low-lives because they can't afford health insurance."

"Let's not worry about Brian now. Dry your hands, and I'll put a Band- Aid on your finger. Then, I'll draw your blood. After that, I'll catch Ms. Krieger before she leaves and get more blood from her. "

Carrie sat on the examining table and held out her arm for Danielle to stick the needle into her vein. "Having you do this to me feels so strange, Dani," she said. "But, at least you're good at it. I've never seen you not get the needle in on the first try."

When Danielle was finished, she squeezed Carrie's hand. "We need to check for Hepatitis B and Hepatitis C, too."

"I've been immunized against Hepatitis B, but I know it's important to check," Carrie said.

Danielle labeled the vials of Carrie's blood. "I'm taking your blood right over to the lab. Now you need to talk to the supervisor. Mrs. Blake is in her office. She'll give you the incident report form. Go right now," Danielle commanded as she left the room.

* * *

Grateful for Dani's calm and professional manner, Carrie composed herself before going to the supervisor's office. Mrs. Blake, a kindly middle- aged woman with salt and pepper gray hair, was busy at her computer when Danielle entered. Stacks of patient charts were piled on a small table beside her.

"Sit down, Carrie," she said, pointing to a chair in front of her desk.

Carrie swallowed hard as she lowered herself into the seat. "I need an incident report. I stuck myself with dirty needle and…." The words came tumbling out until all Mrs. Blake's questions had been answered.

"These things happen," the supervisor said. "You've been here nearly two years, Carrie, and your evaluations have been excellent. You're an intelligent and caring nurse, a credit to the profession. We'll follow up on this, do all we can for you."

Carrie wished Mrs. Blake's complimentary words could comfort her, but talking about her mistake only made her feel more fearful and disgusted with herself.

She sat in Mrs. Blake's office for over an hour completing the paperwork. She documented everything about her health, from childhood illnesses up to the birth control pills she now took. Even though she had no significant health problems, she felt as exposed as if she were standing naked on the center stage of a large lecture hall.

Later that afternoon, Carrie's blood test results came back from the lab; the report read no evidence of HIV or hepatitis. She hadn't been worried about the first test. That one was to make sure she didn't already have an HIV infection or AIDS.

Ms. Krieger's lab results were a different story. Her report showed the continued presence of HIV antibodies but no evidence of hepatitis.

Danielle and Mrs. Blake went with Carrie to see the health department physician, Dr. Majors. He prescribed two antiretroviral medications to prevent a possible HIV infection and gave her a week's worth of samples to give her time to see her primary physician.

Once the nurses were back in Mrs. Blake's office, Danielle handed Carrie a paper cup filled with water and ordered, "Start them now; the sooner the better."

Carrie's hand shook as she put the pills in her mouth and lifted the cup to her lips.

She squeezed her eyes closed as she swallowed them.

Mrs. Blake hugged her. "Go home, Carrie. You've had more than enough excitement for today."

* * *

On the drive home, dormant memories of her Uncle Rick swept over her in waves. He was an actor, gay, and only thirty years old when he died of complications from AIDS. She'd been fourteen years old at the time. At first, her parents wouldn't tell her what made him sick and refused to let her visit; but when she put up enough of a fuss, they relented. Then they explained the disease to her and taught her the importance of hand wash- ing and following 'universal precautions'. She was scared when she first walked into his apartment and saw him, gaunt and weak, lying in a hospital bed. That night she cried for hours and promised herself she would visit him at least once a week. She kept her promise even though it became more difficult, because Rick grew weaker and weaker. Talking to the different home health care nurses who took care of him softened the pain she felt seeing him so helpless.

His words right before he died comforted her through the funeral and the weeks beyond. "Sweetheart, I've had a good life and the best nurses in the world. You can't imagine what a difference they've made these last months. They're helping me die with peace and grace; dignity, too. If it weren't for them, I don't know what I'd do. I understand why people call nurses 'angels on earth'."

Uncle Rick's words stuck with Carrie all through high school. When it came time for her to choose a career, there was no question in her mind what she would pick. After she graduated from nursing school, she worked one year in a hospital and then took this job working in the health department's primary care clinic.

* * *

Brian's SUV stood in the driveway when she arrived home. Thoughts of how and when she would tell him, or even if she would tell him, flooded her mind. As she opened the car door, she wiped the tears from her face and braced herself. Telling Brian wasn't going to be easy. She couldn't guarantee him that she wouldn't become HIV positive.

He sat in front of the television watching a baseball game. She tossed her purse on the coffee table and sat beside him on the sofa.

He took her hand and pressed it to his lips. "I'm sorry about last night. I was a jerk." His eyes remained fixed on the screen as he watched a runner being thrown out on second.

"I'm sorry I lost it, too. I do love my job, and I know I forget about time; but I love you more." The words that came out of her mouth weren't the words she wanted to say. She could tell him about the needle stick after dinner, after the ball game. She snuggled close to him. He slid his arm around her waist and began caressing her, moving his hand up and down her back. Then his other hand reached for her breasts. When he turned to kiss her, she knew she couldn't wait any longer.

"I got stuck with a needle today," she blurted.

He raised his head. "So?"

She pulled back from him and turned her face away. "The patient has AIDS."

He leaned into the pillow on the sofa, rested his legs on the coffee table, and then picked up a glass of beer from the end table. "That was clumsy of you."

"It was an accident. This is serious, Brian. Can you turn the TV off, so I can explain?"

"It's the eighth inning! Four to three. Can't it wait another ten minutes?" He thumped his feet to the floor and leaned forward.

She grabbed the remote control and pushed the off button. "I have to take medication for a bit, probably four weeks. Just as a precaution!" she added when his eyes widened in alarm, either from her effrontery at turning off the television or her news, she didn't know.

"God. I told you to quit that damned job last winter. You go to work to take care of sick people and bring every freaking germ home with you. How many colds did I catch because of you? And now AIDS! Is that what you're telling me? You could have AIDS? No way, Baby. I'm not hanging around for a month waiting to get sick from you again, not with AIDS."

"That's not how it works, Brian," she pleaded. "Listen to me. I'll be all right. I'm taking the medicine just as a precaution. We need to talk. Let me explain."

"No." He held his hands out as if warding off the devil himself. "I'm going to my brother's. I've got to think. I can't deal with all this now."

"Brian! I need you. What happened to 'for better or worse, in sickness and in health'? We said those words to each other two years ago. Please stay." She reached her hand out to him, but he backed further toward the door.

"I'll pick up my things later. This is the last straw, Carrie."

Stunned by his complete rejection and the possible consequences of her actions, Carrie threw herself across their bed and cried herself into a restless sleep. In a vivid dream, she saw herself draped in a shroud, lying in a wooden coffin beside the decomposing body of her Uncle Rick. She awoke in a sweat, her body trembling, and she curled up in a ball and hugged her knees to her chest. She wished her mother were still alive, so she could talk to her. She longed for daylight; life would seem less frightening. As the dawn light filtered through her window, she fell into a deep slumber only to be awakened by her alarm clock at seven-thirty. Mrs. Blake had told her to stay home today, but she wanted to be there. She needed the comfort of her caring coworkers. Talking to clients and the routine of work would keep her busy and her mind off herself.

At the clinic, she put up a good front against her fears, declaring she wasn't worried and pushing last night's argument with Brian to the back of her mind. By the end of the day, with Danielle and Mrs. Blake's encouraging support, she had almost forgotten yesterday's traumas.

When she arrived home, she was surprised to see Brian's car once again in the driveway and Brian himself waiting for her at the door. "I've come back," he said simply, offering no apology.

"I can see that," she answered with a cool glare in her eyes. "What changed your mind?"

"I really do love you, Carrie. I discussed your problem with my brother, and he agrees that I ought to be here for you. We just can't have sex for six months until we're sure that you're not-um-positive."

She slammed her purse down on the kitchen counter. "Brian, you don't know anything. We can have sex using condoms."

"But Tom said..."

"Tom's not a doctor. Either you're with me in this, Brian, or you're not.

Which is it?" she shouted.

"Look, I know he's not a doctor. And I'm not a nurse either, thank God."

"What's that supposed to mean?" She opened the fridge and yanked out a package of chicken breasts and a bag of frozen broccoli to cook for dinner.

"You're the one always trying to cure the world. I can't be that way. I don't want to be that way. I design computer programs."

"That nobody understands."

"At least they're logical. Don't bother fixing me anything. I'll have cold pizza."

The next evening he relented and helped her prepare supper. In the days that followed, they settled into a routine of cooking, eating, television, then bed. He kept to his side; she to hers until the medication began to give her side effects.

She woke up one night with nausea, painful cramps and diarrhea that persisted into the morning making her late for work. The next night, she moved into the den to sleep.

By the end of the month, she'd lost seven pounds. Brian didn't remark on the change in her appearance.

He remained sullen and withdrawn.

* * *

In six weeks, Danielle drew Carrie's blood again. Later, Mrs. Blake called Carrie into her office. She smiled and said, "Your blood test came back negative for HIV antibodies."

"Thank God," Carrie whispered. "I'm so relieved. It's been the longest six weeks of my life."

"That makes two of us," Mrs. Blake said. She stepped toward Carrie and hugged her.

Elated with the news, she rushed home to tell Brian. He shrugged his shoulders and said, "That's great. We can wait a little longer though before we get back together. We should be absolutely sure you're safe."

"Fine," she said. Her feelings were hurt yet again, but this time she wasn't going to give him the satisfaction of begging. She continued to sleep in the den. During the past six weeks, she'd slowly moved nearly all her belongings in there anyway, and she was getting used to sleeping on the futon.

One evening she was brushing her hair before getting under the blankets on the futon when Brian knocked on her doorframe. "I need to talk to you."

"So come in and talk."

He stepped inside and took a deep breath, like a kid getting ready to recite a poem in school. "I want to get my own apartment for a while."

She lowered the hand holding the hairbrush and stared at him. She knew sleeping apart had been troublesome to him, but she hadn't thought their relationship had deteriorated that much. "You want to move out?" Her voice cracked.

"Yeah, I do. I've been giving this a lot of thought. In there." He pointed to their bedroom door. "I want kids."

"So do I, Brian." She stood up. "Before we got married, we both wanted four children. Remember how the minister lectured us on getting to know each other better before we had them? How he said a strong marriage…" She choked on the words and couldn't continue. She began to cry.

"He never said anything about AIDS. There's nothing more I can do here." She took a step toward him.

"Look at you," he said pointing at her.

She looked down to see that her robe had fallen open exposing her body.

"Your damned ribs are sticking out."

"Brian, please don't leave. We have so much to look forward to." He turned his back and stormed into the master bedroom.

* * *

Brian didn't get his own apartment, but he did move back in with his brother. A week later, after no contact, he showed up again on her doorstep.

"I can't live without you, it seems." He hugged her gently, and Carrie felt her heart glow with happiness. He was home. Unfortunately, the honeymoon didn't last long. Within days, they were at each other's throats again. He accused her of being more interested in her patients than in him and not helping him get through the 'AIDS crisis', as he called it. She blamed him for being self-centered and obsessive.

"That does it! We're going to counseling, Brian," she announced one evening when he once again brought up the subject of never having children because of her carelessness in getting stuck with a needle.

The therapist helped them create a kind of truce where they only discussed serious issues in her office where she could run interference. In spite of all the talking, Brian still refused to return to an intimate relationship.

Her three-month blood check again proved to be negative for HIV antibodies, and the two of them went out to celebrate. Whether it was the relief or the wine, Carrie didn't care. Brian wouldn't let her go to the den that night, and they resumed a normal sexual relationship. Carrie thought her marital problems had ended.

By this time, Carrie had regained the weight she had lost from the medication side effects. The two of them resumed their discussions about starting a family. They decided that Carrie would stop taking the birth control pills, hoping that she might get pregnant quickly.

* * *

She felt strong, happy and confident when Danielle drew the blood for the fourth time. The next afternoon Carrie was finishing up with her last patient. As she was putting away her supplies, a health department clerk gave her a message that Mrs. Blake needed to see her right away. Carrie swallowed hard as she opened her supervisor's office door. "It's bad news, isn't it?" she said.

Mrs. Blake had tears in her eyes. "Yes, this blood test showed the presence of HIV antibodies."

Carrie grabbed a bookend from her supervisor's desk and sent it crashing to the floor where it shattered into small shreds. Then, she collapsed in a chair. "Why? Why? Why me? What did I ever do? One lousy needle prick in the finger. One!" She leaned forward, her eyes pleading for understanding from Mrs. Blake. "The odds are against it. I was doing so well. Why?"

Mrs. Blake ignored the marble shreds on the floor. "I know, Honey. I know. And you're right. It's unusual to have three negatives and then a positive; but it happens. You'll have to be careful."

"Now I'll need to get a confirmation test, the Western Blot," Carrie said through her tears. "Will this never end?"

Mrs. Blake put her arms around Carrie. "We'll do the Western Blot now. Take some time off work, as long as you need. This whole thing has been a nightmare for us all."

Carrie, still in shock, slumped back into the chair. "I'm quitting, Mrs. Blake. I'm done working here. The job's ruining my marriage, my life. Maybe later, when and if this is ever over, I'll go back to nursing, a desk job though." She gave a little laugh. "Maybe with an insurance company, telephone triage, or something like that."

Mrs. Blake took a deep breath. "For now, Danielle will draw your blood again. Then go home and rest. Try to relax. Stay home 'til you feel better." Her voice cracked.

"Relax! I wish!"

"I hope you change your mind about quitting. We love you here. You're a natural community health nurse. I pray this test result was a mistake. You're still on the payroll for the rest of the month whether you're here or not."

Carried murmured, "thank you." She was exhausted; her legs felt like lead, much too heavy to lift to take a step. Dani had suggested taking Brian out to a restaurant to tell him the bad news, but she didn't have the heart or the energy for it. They'd been doing so well lately; his attitude seemed to have changed. Surely he'd understand that they could get through this together. At dinner she broke the news to him. They were sitting at the kitchen table eating chicken and dumplings, one of Brian's favorite meals. He was quiet; his eyes staring in disbelief. She ended the little speech she had rehearsed with, "I handed in my resignation today. I'll never go back there again, Brian. I promise. No more needles to stick into myself. I'll take the medicine. I'll be all right."

"The hell you will. I'm not going to sit here and watch you die. I've been through this once with you, remember?" He pushed his food away and left the table.

"Where are you going?"

"Back to Tom's. And this time, don't expect me back. We'll be over tomorrow to get my stuff. I want the big screen TV. You can have the portable. You're never home to watch TV anyway."

"According to you, I'll be dying. I won't have anything else to do except watch TV." She followed him down the hall to the bedroom. "Brian, we have to talk."

He turned quickly and grabbed a suitcase from the closet and stuffed the clothes from his dresser into it, then filled a duffel bag with his underwear and CDs. Carrie watched him, disbelieving. Always before he only took a few things, enough to get by for a few days. When he was finished, he pushed past her and walked out the front door without saying anything more.

* * *

Three days later, Carrie received a registered letter from an attorney's office. With shaking fingers, she opened it to find official separation papers. An attached letter advised her to contact her own attorney and sign an agreement for an amicable separation, which would end in divorce a year from the date of signing.

"No one to blame, except me," she said to herself, remembering the pinprick from the dirty needle.

She sat on a kitchen stool and looked around the room. How would she support herself if she did have full blown AIDS? With her period three weeks late, was she pregnant or just overstressed? Already her breasts were full and tender. She'd need to get a pregnancy kit at the drug store. Who would be there for her, or her and the baby? Should she get an abortion?

Everything would depend on the results of the Western Blot. She picked up the telephone to call Dani when she heard a knock at the door. Hoping that it might be Brian changing his mind, she dropped the phone and ran to fling the door open, but it was only the *FedEx* man with a special delivery. She signed the form on the clipboard, and he handed her a large cardboard envelope.

Her first thought was to toss it in the trash, since it probably was a follow-up from Brian or his lawyer about their 'amicable separation.' She felt so nauseated at the moment that she didn't want to read anything from anybody. She dragged herself back to the kitchen and ripped the envelope open. Inside was a regular business sized envelope. The return address was the lab where her blood had been tested. "What do they want now?" She tore that one and pulled out a report.

Your blood test of September 21, 2012 was a false positive for HIV antibodies, an error. The second analysis, the Western Blot, was also negative for HIV antibodies. Therefore, your blood shows no evidence of an HIV infection. We're sorry for any inconvenience this may have caused you.

NEITHER HERE NOR THERE

The dedicated life is the life worth living.
Annie Dillard

Jahan Hazzare leaned on his daughter's arm as he stared at the headstone of his wife's grave. "My beautiful Chandni, how can I leave her here in this cold ground? I should have returned her to her homeland, back to New Delhi. She always wanted to die there. Instead she grows this ugly thing in her brain."

His daughter corrected him. "An astrocytoma, *Pitaa*. And you aren't the only one who misses Mom."

He pulled away from her. "I know very well what it was, Tapati!" He realized his anger shouldn't be directed at his daughter, but he felt such a failure as a doctor and as a husband for not being able to save his wife's life. "Come live with Anthony and me, *Pitaa*," Tapati asked as they walked back to the cemetery parking lot.

A damp November wind blew dead leaves from the maple trees down to the ground where they swirled eerily around the rows of headstones. "*Mitaa* would have wanted it. Taking care of family is the Indian way. You've told me that since I've been a little girl."

Anthony, Tapati's husband, chimed in, "You can have the entire west wing of our house. We'll all eat dinner together, and you can spend the evenings with us."

Jahan ran his hand over his eyes. "I want to keep my place, the house Tapati grew up in. I've lived there for thirty-two years. I can still take care of it. I admit, it's overwhelming at times, but I can do it."

"We want you with us now. We wished both you and *Mitaa* had come when she first got sick."

"Ah, Tapati, give me time to think. My Chandni, my beautiful wife. The astrocytoma in her brain. The diagnosis was so unexpected."

Tapati squeezed his arm. "You made sure she had the best care. Dr. Hassad is the top neurosurgeon in the country."

"It wasn't enough, Tapati. She died soon after the operation, died in my arms. We didn't have a chance to say a final good-bye. All she did at the end was sleep."

Tears filled Jahan's eyes. "Me, a doctor, and I couldn't save her! What good am I?" He picked up the bouquet of roses he had placed on the headstone earlier and fell to his knees, clasping the roses to his chest as if he still held his beloved Chandni. To still be near her was why he wanted a traditional burial and not cremation as most Hindus desire. His one consolation was his belief in karma and reincarnation and that she was one step closer to Nirvana.

"*Pitaa*," Anthony, Jahan's son-in-law said, "No one could have saved her. At the end, you gave her CPR and called 911. The emergency room doctors did everything they could." Anthony took his father-in-law's arm and helped him to the car. "We'll drive you home."

"You're a good boy," Jahan said, patting Anthony's hand. "Let me think more about this move. Your house is big. And it is the

94

Indian way for children to care for their parents when they are old." He rubbed his aching right knee. "It getting harder for me to drive." He settled himself in the back seat.

Jahan glanced at himself in the rear view mirror and saw pain and anger in his dark brown eyes and deep lines across his forehead. When he ran his hand over the top of his bald head, he remembered the thick black wavy hair he once had.

"Anthony, I think about Chandni when we were young, Tapati's age, thirty-two years ago, already. Her *Pitaa* didn't think I was good enough to be her husband, but he gave his permission, even his blessing. He saw we loved each other, just like Tapati loves you. You are like a son to me." He patted Anthony's shoulder.

Andrew looked in his rear view mirror at Jahan slouched in the back seat and gave him a quick grin. "Before marrying Tapati, I was afraid of you. I didn't think you thought I was good enough for her," he said.

"Ah, we from the old country have a lot to learn. I always thought Tapati would marry a Hindu, not an Italian Christian, Catholic no less, like you. We bring our children here and expect them to live like they do in India. In the old country the children are committed to the family, to each other, and to our religion. We never waver. In the United States, we must bend. After all, we live here. America is your world, not India. I didn't know this back then, Anthony, but I do now." Jahan waved his arms as if encircling the globe. "Tapati was right to choose you for her husband."

When Tapati turned around, Jahan saw tears in her eyes. Her shoulder length black hair reminded him so much of Chandni. He had loved the bronze of his wife's skin, her warm smile, and her trim figure. Why did she have to die? He took two white linen handkerchiefs from his lapel pocket and handed one to his daughter. "We will both go back to work on Monday. Me only for a few weeks; you probably for twenty more years. Work is good, Tapati. It keeps your mind off of sadness."

"*Mitaa* would want us to be happy. Let's try, *Pitaa*." Chandni switched the radio on.

Jahan's back ached, and he shifted his position and closed his eyes. Frank Sinatra was singing 'I Did it My Way' from the car's surround-sound stereo. Long forgotten memories of his wife drifted through his mind.

Chandni had been gone eleven months now. If only she were still alive, they could go back to India to live. Why had he insisted Chandni move to America right after they were married? Perhaps it was a mistake to have come to Cleveland to accept the oncology residency forty years ago? His eyes felt heavy. He sighed, suddenly longing for the old country, where he had spent his childhood surrounded by aunts, uncles, and cousins. Tonight, he wished he still lived in India and could relive his memories of the past.

As Anthony parked the automobile in the driveway, Jahan again thought of Chandni. She was usually there to greet him when he came home. Tonight, no one looked out the window watching for him. Slowly, fumbling with the keys in his pocket, he walked up his porch steps. Anthony and Tapati watched from the car until he unlocked the door.

He entered the house, flipped on the overhead light switch, and sank into his recliner.

Tonight there was no smiling face to greet him, no long bear hug, and no *masala* tea and his favorite cheese and split pea dish, *mutter panir*, served with homemade yogurt. And there was no relaxed dinner, which she had served hot, no matter how late he was. Some evenings they ate at ten or eleven. On those days, she served two family suppers, his and an earlier one at six for Tapati.

He remembered her words of comfort when he told her that

he'd lost a patient. "Ah, Jahan, I wish all cancer patients had you for an oncologist. You are compassionate and knowledgeable. The people know it too."

"Sad times like this I wish we could live in India and the United States at the same time," he told Chandni. "There is comfort in the old ways."

"You brought me here, Love. Moving to Cleveland was hard at first, but it's okay now. Tapati is happy here and you are mostly happy, so I am happy, too. Someday we will go back to the homeland."

On the nights he was particularly stressed or discouraged, she rubbed his back.

A lump formed in his throat thinking about her. He looked at the old wedding photos of Tapati and Anthony, dusty now, in frames on the bookshelf and remembered how hesitant he'd been about blessing his daughter's upcoming marriage. How he'd talked to the priest, Father Patel. With shame, he still recalls the day twenty-six years ago, months before Tapati's wedding, when he walked unannounced into the priest's office.

"*Pundit ji,* I need to talk about Tapati and Anthony."

"Still misgivings?"

"Father, Tapati's Anthony is not Indian and not a Hindu. He's Italian and Roman Catholic, a mere accountant, no physician. I wanted my daughter to marry a doctor, someone smart, able to make money, and care about people."

"It's hard to see our children grow up and do things that we don't approve of. Take my advice. Tapati is a smart girl, well-educated with her engineering degree. I've talked to them both. Anthony is a good man. They love each other. Give your blessing to this marriage."

Jahan followed the priest's advice and gracefully blessed the marriage. After the wedding, Jahan forced himself to embrace Anthony as his son. "We're family now, Anthony," he reluctantly told the young man. "I will be a father to you. You're one of us now. The Indian network connections will be here for you. It's our way."

Anthony swallowed hard. "And I will be there for you, *Pitaa*, be your and Chandni's son."

When the water pipes broke, it was Anthony he called. He came right away and spent half the night fixing them. Jahan was not a handyman yet he hated to give repairmen his money, unless they were from India, of course, so this arrangement pleased him. In time Anthony took over the finances of the oncology practice, something Jahan never had time for either. Under Anthony's management, the profits increased.

Anthony set up a computer at home and showed him how to receive and send e-mails so he could communicate with his family in New Delhi. Maybe moving in with them would work out in a year or so. Now his thoughts centered on retirement.

After all, he was seventy-two and fighting rheumatoid arthritis and early emphysema. But what would he do in retirement? He didn't know. He'd dedicated his life to medicine and had few other interests. It was a work he loved and one that helped him make sense out of life.

Later in the month, he reluctantly informed his partners that he'd be closing his practice within a month. They shook his hand and congratulated him on his decision. Jahan sensed the office would get along fine without him. He was pleased to learn a young Indian doctor who he respected would take his place.

During his retirement dinner at his favorite Indian restaurant, *The Needlam,* his physician friends told humorous yet poignant stories about his career. How he'd managed a ten-year-old leukemia patient's chemotherapy. The afternoon he spent hours counseling an estranged family so that the children were able to make peace with their mother before she died. And the time he slipped in the hospital hallway on spilled coffee, quickly stood up, and grabbed the mop from the janitor's hands to clean the floor himself.

When the emcee handed him the microphone, he could hardly speak, he was so overwhelmed. "Thank you, thank you...." His voice cracked, and tears filled his eyes.

Anthony helped him down from the podium back to his chair.

Once the emptiness of retirement set in, Jahan felt useless. For several weeks, he drove by his old office but never had the courage to go in and inquire how his former patients were doing. Instead he read the *Journal of the American Medical Association* from cover to cover and watched the ups and downs of the stock market on CNBC.

Several weeks later, hoping he would be happier with his family around, he told Tapati and Anthony he would sell his house and move in with them.

He could tell they were pleased.

"Finally *Pitaa*," Tapati said. Anthony smiled. "Now there will be two men in the house."

Tapati and Andrew found a realtor to list his home; it sold in less than a month. The couple helped him organize an estate sale, manage the paper work of the house sale, and move his bedroom furniture and personal belongings into their home.

To his surprise, he discovered he was even more depressed living at his daughter's, yet he presented an acceptable facade for friends and acquaintances. At night, he often lay awake in bed thinking of Chandni and how they used to sleep snuggled together like two spoons.

He remembered Trish, Chandni's home care nurse, and how she made those last weeks of her life bearable for him. She didn't manage the medications or the clinical part of his wife's care; Jahan and her doctor did that. Trish focused on the emotional and comfort piece that he so needed. He wished he had someone like her in his life. He thought about contacting her but felt too embarrassed to make the call.

Both Tapati and Anthony left for work before seven in the morning and didn't return home until after six.

As the weeks passed, Jahan began staying in bed until eleven in the morning and reluctantly got out of bed feeling groggy and unsteady. Soon he quit reading his journal and sat in a recliner mesmerized by the television. His appetite was poor, and he lost twelve pounds in several months. The stiffness in his legs scared him; it was almost impossible for him to walk up and down steps now or get in and out of a car by himself. Tapati made an appointment with the doctor.

His rheumatologist started him on a new medication and prescribed in-home physical therapy.

Jahan followed his exercise regimen carefully. "It's hard work to grow stronger. Maybe the Hindu gods will help me," he told the physical therapist.

Anthony set up a *puja*, a private prayer shrine, in their home for Jahan, as it was now too difficult to drive the old man to the temple every day. Only with Tapati and Anthony's help could Jahan attend the service.

Tapati tried to pay her father extra attention. Because of her ten-hour day work schedule and disinterest in cooking Indian food, Jahan complained.

"You are not like your mother. You have lost many of the Indian ways. You are of the 'half in, half out' generation."

Tapati bit her lip. "I'm sorry. I feel bad about that, *Pitaa*."

She attempted the more complex Indian recipes Chandni used

to make, *makai simla mirch*, corn and green bell pepper curry, and *khumb matar masala*, curried mushrooms with peas.

"Nothing tastes right. Even the *mutter panir* you cook is too soft and the *chapati* flat bread is too heavy," Jahan complained.

As time passed, Jahan became more cranky and demanding, delivered political diatribes about the Mideast wars and the deteriorating health care system, and accused Anthony of mismanaging his money. He refused take the antidepressants his physician prescribed.

Tapati told Anthony, "We must accept his difficult behavior. That's what happens to older people, what we can expect. It's normal in our culture. We still must honor him."

Anthony replied, "Of course. I'll feel the same about my parents when they'll need help."

"India's the best place on earth," Jahan told Anthony as they sat in the living room drinking masala tea after dinner. "I want to go back, see my nieces and nephews and visit the old town outside New Delhi."

"It'll be a long flight," Anthony said. "India will be different now, not like you remember it."

Jahan set his tea cup on the coffee table. "I'll go alone if you and Tapati won't go with me."

For weeks, Jahan persisted in his threat. Finally, thinking it might ease his depression, Tapati and Andrew relented, agreeing to a two-week visit.

The trip was a struggle. The wheelchair they ordered didn't have footrests. The fast pace of the airport confused Jahan, and he complained about needing to be buckled in his seat while the plane was in the air. When they arrived in New Delhi, Jahan's niece had arranged for a driver to pick them up at the airport.

"I want to drive myself. I don't need a chauffeur," Jahan told

Anthony.

"Look at the cars. The drivers are crazy. It's been a long time since you drove on the left side. Let the taxi take us. Your niece already paid the Rai's for this service."

He sighed. "All right."

After Anthony helped him into the cab's passenger seat, Jahan sat back and closed his eyes. He looked out the window, his mind already diverted.

"You see how they respect the cows, Anthony? They would never do this in the United States, permit cows to amble down the street without fear of injury. Cows are revered and considered sacred here; people protect them. We don't kill them and eat them like in America."

"I know, *Pitaa*. You have told me that many times."

"And people are everywhere, but few rush like people do in America. Look at the cute little monkeys scrambling around in the trees." He pointed to an older gentleman on the sidewalk. "See the monkey sitting on that man's shoulders. A minute ago, he leaped down and stole food right from his fingers."

Tapati shook her head. "Let's hope no monkey steals our food."

* * *

Their driver took them to a small two-bedroom country house, a three hour drive outside the city, where Jahan's niece lived with her husband and four children. Tears ran down his cheeks when he saw his Indian family. "My God, why did I ever leave? It makes no sense to me now."

His niece hugged him. "We lost track of you, *Chacha*, but you were always in our hearts. Come. Relax in the chair by the window."

Once he sat down, Jahan yawned and rubbed his forehead.

His niece walked over to take his arm. "Come, *Chacha*. I'll show you where you will sleep"

Anthony carried Jahan's suitcase into his bedroom. "Rest, *Pitaa*. It is late. Tomorrow is another day."

The next morning Jahan cornered Anthony in the hallway. "The house is drafty. I go to sleep cold and wake up cold. I must wear a sweater all the time," he muttered.

After breakfast, he pushed his chair back from the table and looked at his niece. "I want my morning shower. My hair feels greasy. I must stink. I haven't had a bath for two days," Jahan complained.

"Tap water is only available in the evenings and early in the morning," his niece told him.

"Oh, I forgot about the water situation. I'll wait until tonight then."

Later Jahan pulled Tapati aside. "The dishes are dirty. There is no soap to wash them, just rinsing them in water is not sanitary."

Tapati ran her hand across her forehead. "This is how you grew up, *Pitaa*."

"Yes, but I feel different now. It's pleasant here, but it drives me crazy at the same time. The pace of life is too slow. I'm bored. All we do is sit around and drink tea. In America, I had a purpose to my life."

People congregated outdoors, kids played in the street, and neighbors exchanged friendly words, but Jahan became more unhappy. "I'm not used to having all these people milling around. I don't like New Delhi any more. I want to go back to Ohio."

Tapati persuaded him to stay the full two weeks. On the day they were to return home, he refused to dress for the flight. As he boarded the aircraft in a gray sweat suit, he told the flight attendant. "I love India. It's the best place in the world." He pointed to Tapati and Anthony. "They're forcing me to go to the United States. They won't let me stay in my own country."

Tapati apologized to the stewardess. "He's been begging to leave for days."

Jahan sat quietly on the plane for the return trip, sleeping, leafing through the travel magazines, watching movies, and slowly walking back and forth to the bathroom, when the 'fasten seatbelt' sign was off. He tapped his foot up and down as the plane landed. "I can't wait to get off," he told Anthony.

* * *

As they drove home from the airport and pulled into their driveway, Jahan said, "It is good to be home. The United States is my country."

Tapati and Anthony looked at each other and sighed.

Three months after their return, Jahan told Anthony, "India is better than America. I will talk to my niece about moving to New Delhi, to finish my days. I'll open an oncology practice there."

Anthony winked at Tapati, then said to Jahan, "You haven't worked for almost six years. The United States has been your home for over forty years, *Pitaa*. We are your family. You need to be with us."

"I don't like living here anymore. I'm not needed here. I'm neither here nor there. I want to go back to my roots."

"Stay with us, *Pitaa*. This is your country now," Anthony counseled. "We will take care of you; we love you." Even Tapati's tears and pleas didn't change his mind.

The couple agreed to a second visit, "Just for him to see India again.

We'll only go for one week this time," Tapati said.

Because of work commitments, Anthony was unable to take this trip. He drove them to the airport and hugged them both goodbye. As Jahan was walking down the ramp to board the plane, he turned to look at Tapati standing beside him. He felt tired and confused, not sure if he should walk back into the airport, not sure that he wanted to go to India after all.

He felt his heart beating fast and pressed his fingers to his wrist. One hundred eight. He must calm down. Tapati would not be sitting with him; the plane was too full. Jahan seat was 11B; hers was 21B. At the end of the ramp, Jahan turned and lifted his hand weakly to wave at Anthony, then remembered that Anthony was still in the airport. He took Tapati's arm and boarded the plane.

* * *

Jahan fidgeted in his seat and rubbed his chest when they were flying over the Arabian Sea. He pressed the 'Help' button.

"I'd like some milk, something for heartburn," he told the flight attendant.

"Are you all right?" she asked.

"Just a little heartburn. Milk will clear it up. I've had it before. While you're here, would you get a pillow and my cell phone from the overhead bin?"

"Here's the phone. You can't use it until we land. I'll prop the pillow behind you and be right back with your milk."

Jahan squeezed the phone in his hand. With fumbling fingers, he tried to press the numbers to call Anthony.

His seatmate stared at him. "You can't make a call now. You heard what the flight attendant told you."

Jahan nodded. Yet he picked up the phone and without dialing, whispered, "Goodbye, Anthony. You are the son I never had. I love you."

He gasped for breath and felt sweat on his brow. The cell phone dropped to the floor. His seatmate pushed the 'Help' button.

Jahan's mental fog temporarily lifted, and he saw Tapati standing over him. Her face looked twisted and misshapen, like he was looking at her distorted image in an amusement park mirror.

He wondered what all the commotion was about. The man holding his wrist, Tapati telling him to 'hang on,' the seatmate getting up and standing in the aisle. When Jahan heard Tapati say, "We're going to land in Bombay and get you in a hospital, he realized he was dying. Not heartburn but a heart attack, that was what had been wrong with him. His world went suddenly black.

* * *

The plane made an emergency landing in the Bombay airport, and an ambulance rushed Jahan, now unconscious, to the hospital. Tapati stayed by his side while he was being treated in the emergency room. "He's my dad, a doctor, an oncologist. Make sure he gets the best care."

He was rushed into the operating room for open heart surgery. Three vessels in his heart were blocked.

Three weeks later, Jahan, though feeble, had recovered enough to be flown back home.

Anthony welcomed him with a big bear hug. "There will be no nursing home for Jahan, I will take some time off work to help," he told Tapati.

At first, Jahan rallied, then another heart attack reduced his cardiac function so severely that he could barely move without becoming short of breath. Severe congestive heart failure, the visiting physician said.

Trish, once Chandni's home health care nurse, was assigned to the case.

"Ah, Trish, it's so good to see you," Jahan said when she

visited him for the first time. He allowed her to listen to his heart and lungs, something he never would have thought possible in his earlier years.

"We're going to get you better, Jahan, just like you helped your patients fight cancer. Physical and occupational therapy for sure."

He took a deep breath. "It's hard work getting stronger. Maybe the Hindu gods will help."

Trish taught Tapati and Anthony about Jahan's medications and ways to keep comfortable. Every day Tapati, Anthony, or a home health aide bathed, diapered, fed, and turned him. They exercised his arms and legs and used a Hoyer Lift to transfer him from his bed to the wheelchair, where he sat almost as still as a statue looking out the window or watching television.

Anthony rubbed his legs when they became cold and shaved him every morning before he went to work. Anthony was the only one who could make Jahan laugh with his 'knock knock' jokes and DVD collection of old Abbott and Costello movies. He read him the *Veda* and amused him by helping him assemble jigsaw puzzles. Some afternoons, he spoon fed Jahan sips of *Kingfish* beer.

"Promise you will take care of Tapati," Jahan begged Anthony one night.

Anthony put his hand on his father-in-law's forehead. "I adore her. She's the love of my life, my family. I wouldn't have it any other way." Anthony tears fell on Jahan's cheek.

Tapati and Anthony took turns sitting with him during the last days of his life. Anthony took the midnight to six a.m. shift. The night before Jahan's seventy-ninth birthday, he lay in bed with pillows propped behind his back, listening to Anthony recite Hindu prayers. Moonlight shone through the window outlining Anthony's face, giving it a soft glow.

Tears came to Jahan's eyes. "You are my son. You make me

feel like I am back in India." For an instant, his eyes bore into Anthony's and locked in a place outside time or space. He reached for his son-in-law's hand.

"*Pitaa*, you are my father."

Seconds later, he felt his daughter's head on his chest and her warm tears on his skin.

Then, Jahan faded into darkness, Anthony and Tapati by his side. Just the three of them. No one else. That was how he wanted it.

Soon a bright light engulfed him and drew him upward. In its center was the faint silhouette of Chandni standing in front of the Taj Mahal.

GOING TO THE DOGS

There are only two creatures of value on the face of the earth: those with the commitment, and those who require the commitment of others.

John Adams

This is the happiest day of my life," Jonathan said the day he married Marie. They sealed the ceremony with a kiss and agreed they'd be together forever. He especially liked the lines in the vows 'to respect, love, cling to each other for better or worse, in sickness and in health as long as they lived.' Knowing he always would have Marie by his side gave him a new sense of security.

Once they were married, Marie wanted to quit her job at the bank, and he readily agreed. His income would be sufficient to support them both. And he didn't mind when she told him she didn't want any children. Neither did he. It was all he could do to take care of himself, and now her.

In the few weeks they'd known each other before the wedding, he hadn't learned a great deal about Marie's past, except that she'd had an abortion in her late teens. It was enough that she was affectionate and caring and seemed to love his Golden Lab, Alexander, almost as much as she loved him.

He had told her about his modest one bedroom house in

Atlanta's suburbs with its little patch of lawn and two red rose bushes.

She said, "It will be perfect, Jonathan, just what I've always wanted."

Marie read the sports pages to him in the mornings while he ate his breakfast. Every day when he came home from work, she rubbed his back and served him a three-course meal. After dinner, holding hands like the young lovers they were, they walked Alexander before going to bed.

And every night before falling asleep, Jonathan held her close and said, "Forever, Darling. Forever together. Sleep well."

Within months, Marie had taken over the household bills, managed all their appointments, and chatted happily about the soap operas she'd watched on television while he worked. Jonathan enjoyed his position as a disability counselor with the state of Georgia. He'd been there for ten years and hoped to retire from the job in another twenty. Then, he and Marie could be together all the time. 'Course by then, he'd have a new dog, but he'd deal with that when he had to. For now, life was good, and he was happy.

* * *

And so it went for two whole years. But, shortly after their second wedding anniversary, Jonathan's job was phased out. He hated having to go home to tell Marie. When he got off the bus, instead of going straight to the house, he walked all the way around the block. Neighbors greeted him cheerfully, and he found it hard to be polite. Their worlds were secure. He was among the ranks of the unemployed.

He opened his front door, filled with dread, knowing Marie would be terribly disappointed in him. She greeted him with her usual kiss. He smelled pot roast cooking, one of his favorites.

"How did it go today?" she asked, as she did every day.

110

"I'm sorry I'm late." He took off his coat and hung it in the front closet.

"Are you?" she asked. "I didn't notice. I was watching a movie on TV. I put dinner in the slow cooker. We can eat as soon as you're ready."

He made himself comfortable in his favorite recliner and took a deep breath before saying, "Marie, darling, aren't you bored staying home all day and just watching television and cooking? Do you ever think of going back to work?"

"Now, what brought that on?" She stood behind him rubbing his shoulders. Alexander sat by his side.

He couldn't postpone it any longer. He had to tell her. "I lost my job today. I say I was fired; they say I was phased out. Like all of a sudden, I'm not in their radar, never to be seen again." He stood up and continued in a theatrical tone, looking this way and that. "'Did you hear what happened to Jonathan Marks?' 'No, what happened to Jonathan Marks?' 'He was phased out'. 'Poor Jonathan, such a nice guy.' Wonder what he'll do now.'"

He slumped back into his recliner. "That's about all the cut back will mean to my co-workers. It will mean a lot to my clients though. I don't know how they're going to get along without me." Alexander pawed at his leg; Jonathan absent-mindedly petted him.

Marie wiped a tear from his face. "It's not so terrible. The state's constantly making budget cuts. We'll get by until we find you another job."

"Don't you think you could go back to work for a while? Banks always want tellers. Even part time."

Marie sat across from him. "I've got enough to do with the house and the yard. We agreed I'd take over those chores, so you wouldn't have to worry about them anymore, and you'd bring in the money. Which I've been managing for you quite nicely, by the way. Between your unemployment and what I've saved, we're good for six months at least. And besides, I decided I might like to have a baby."

This news shocked Jonathan. "You said you didn't want children. You implied that the abortion made pregnancy impossible!"

"I didn't mean to give you that impression, Jon. But I'm nearly thirty-one. My time for having kids is running out. If we have a baby and don't like it, we can always give it up for adoption. On TV, I saw a lady who dropped hers off on the hospital steps."

Those comment struck him as outlandish, but never having been married and not dating much before meeting Marie, he supposed women could be peculiar when it came to babies and hormonal changes. He'd worked with enough female clients to know that much.

"You're not already pregnant, are you?" he asked, praying for a negative response.

"Don't be silly. I'm still on the pill. A baby's just something I'm thinking about."

Staying home with Marie all day was a revelation to Jonathan. She still leaped out of bed to cook him a full breakfast and read him the sport's pages from the morning newspaper. At the time he would normally leave for work, she began her daily routine, which wasn't really a routine at all. Some days she sat and watched television at full volume and other days, she raced through her cleaning chores, dusting, laundry, and running the vacuum. Those days she put him in the mind of a whirling dervish.

Weeks went by with no luck in his job search. Even with Marie helping, he had only one interview in four months. Feeling like a failure, he became depressed and hated that Marie was stuck married to him, but she seemed fine. She went out and did the grocery shopping at *Wal-Mart* instead of the specialty shops and brought home *McDonald's* instead of them going out to eat at nice restaurants. The more cheerful she acted, the more miser- able he became. Her shopping trips began to last longer and longer, so that frequently he had to walk Alexander in the evenings by himself. The neighbors asked the same question, "Find anything yet, Jonathan?"

"Not yet."

"We'll keep our eyes opened for you. Kind of difficult when you're so specialized."

"I know," he'd respond and walk on, head down, around the block, and back into his little house, hoping that Marie would be home standing by the stove. Even in their reduced circumstances, Marie could cook up a mean meal.

Out of the blue, six months after he'd been laid off, Jonathan arrived home from his walk to Marie's cheerful outburst. "We have to get a puppy."

"A puppy? Why a puppy? Alexander is only six years old." He bent down to ruff the top of Alexander's head, as if to reassure the dog he wouldn't be replaced anytime soon.

"I decided I don't want a baby. This house is way too small. But, it isn't too small for a puppy. That way I can have a dog of my own, like you have Alexander. And I can buy clothes and jewelry for it. God knows, you spend more time with that animal than you do with me anymore. You never hold me like you used to; we don't go out. It's all so boring."

"If you're so bored, maybe you should go back to work," Jonathan said more harshly than he intended. He loved Marie; she was his life.

"Maybe I will," she said, then added, "And maybe I won't. What's it to you anyway?"

The telephone rang. Jonathan had been standing closest to it and picked it up on the first ring.

Marie shrieked, "Don't answer that!" and grabbed the receiver from his hand before he could say anything.

She slammed it down.

"What's wrong with you, Marie?"

"Nothing. I have to go out for a while. I'm going to the park. Don't answer the phone if it rings. No one's going to call about a job this late in the day."

"What about dinner?" he asked. He felt helpless. He didn't know this new woman Marie had become.

"It's on the stove. You can heat it up. You took care of yourself before we got married. You can do it again."

"Marie," he cried in alarm. "You're not leaving me, are you? If you want a baby that badly, we can work something out. Don't leave me, please."

"I'm not leaving you. I'm going to look at a puppy you won't let me have. Just for the fun of it."

She brushed past him. He smelled her cologne and wanted to grab her and take her into the bedroom and make love. But she was gone in a moment.

The phone rang again while he ate his leftover spaghetti. He put his hand on the receiver but hesitated to pick it up. Probably one of those sales calls. That was surely why Marie didn't want him to answer it earlier. The phone kept ringing. He finally picked it up.

"Jonathon, it's Claire, Marie's aunt. I've been trying to contact her for some time. She hasn't returned my calls for a month. I'm worried about her. She's still taking her medicine, isn't she?"

"Medicine?"

114

"You know, for her bi-polar disease. You do know, don't you, Jon?"

"Marie never told me about any bi-polar problem. I don't think she takes medicine for anything. Hardly even takes her daily multi-vitamins."

"This is serious. Can you find out?"

"I'll ask her when she gets home." Jonathan felt too embarrassed to tell Claire he was unemployed and also worried about the recent changes in his wife's behavior.

"Good thing I'm a nurse, Jon. I spent years trying to help her control her roller-coaster emotions and impulsive behavior. Worked on organizing daily activities and setting manageable goals. The new medicines have been a Godsend. When she moved from San Diego, I lined her up with a psychiatrist there in Atlanta. He's been monitoring her medicine."

"Marie is bi-polar? How long?" Jonathan asked, completely shocked that Marie had never talked about her illness. He thought her erratic behavior was related to his being around the house most of the day.

"We found out when she was in high school." Claire started to cry. "If I weren't so old, I'd hop on a plane tomorrow. I love that girl. She's been a challenge though."

"I love her, too." Jonathon rubbed his forehead with the palm of his hand. His voice cracked.

"Jon, I'm so sorry to tell you all this, and I'm sorry I missed the wedding. The doctor said I couldn't take the flight."

"She understood."

"Marie told me she was marrying a counselor, and I assumed you were working with her. My daughter here in California told me she's seen nearly nude photos of Marie with a Back Lab puppy on *Facebook*, the Internet site, you know. Since then, I've been trying to get in touch with her without alarming you. I tried to get hold of her doctor and just learned he's closed his private practice, now he works for the VA, veterans, you know."

"She never talks about a psychiatrist."

"He left his private practice months ago, didn't let me know even though I was paying the bills and Marie had signed the paper for me to stay abreast of her condition. Gross negligence, I'd say. The good part is he never cashed the checks I sent."

Jonathan ran his hand through his hair. "Just left his practice?"

"You of all people must understand. They say his caseload with the HMO was impossible. I admit I let the ball drop by not keeping up."

Jonathan finished his conversation with Claire and returned to his dinner. But he was no longer hungry. At that moment, he didn't care what anyone thought. He slid the food from his plate into Alexander's bowl. The dog slurped noisily at the spaghetti, then sat back down next to Jonathan and burped. Jonathan laughed, in spite of his shock and misery to learn that Marie was probably e-mailing guys on *Facebook*. He and Alexander went into the living room. He turned on the CD player and waited for his wife to come home. He'd really have to talk to her.

Bi-polar! She probably needs strong medications, anti-psychotics, maybe even lithium. No children then.

But perhaps they could have a second dog. Introduce it slowly to the family. Alexander had always been a good-natured creature. Jonathan turned the volume up and leaned back in the recliner. He'd tell her when she came home.

He was half asleep and the music had stopped when Alexander growled. It was the dog's way of letting Jonathan know that someone was walking up his sidewalk. Jonathan sat up with the snap of the recliner and brushed his hair off his forehead. He waited expectantly, prepared to give her the good news about getting a puppy.

The doorbell rang. Puzzled, he got up. Marie probably forgot her key.

He walked to the door and opened it with a smile on his face.

"Mr. Marks? I'm Don Bartlett, Police officer for Ridgewood. May I come in?"

With a sinking feeling, Jonathan stepped aside to let him enter. "Is something wrong?'

"I'm sorry. Perhaps you want to sit down. Can I get you a glass of water?"

"I don't need any water, thank you. What happened? Is it Marie? Is she dead?" Jonathan fumbled his way back to his recliner, Alexander by his side.

"No, Sir. No. She's not dead. The driver of the car is though. A William Connors. A friend of yours?"

Jonathan stiffened. "No, never heard of him. My wife was with him. Is that what you're trying to tell me?"

The policeman cleared his throat. "Yes, Sir. Marie's been taken to Memorial Hospital. I can drive you there if you like. She's been seriously injured. They had to do emergency surgery. You might want to be with her when she wakes up. The doctor first thought she might lose her vision. Severe head trauma."

Jonathan felt bile rise up in his throat. He forced himself to swallow, then reached for the handle of Alexander's guide harness.

"I have to get Alexander ready to go. Come, Boy."

"I'm sorry, Sir. You can't take your dog." The officer stopped.

"Alexander's always at my side. I can't go outside without him. He's been my eyes for six years now."

Once the dog was outfitted in his harness, Jonathan stood, the dog at his side, ready to go to the hospital to comfort Marie. After all, he promised, 'for better or worse, in sickness and in health.'

BURNING THE MIDNIGHT OIL

*People are like stained glass windows. They sparkle and shine
when the sun is out, but when the darkness sets in, their true
beauty is revealed only if there is a light from within.*

Elizabeth Kubler-Ross

I love Brenda's lamp. From my kitchen window, I can see it,
this antique lamp of my neighbor's. The way it sits on her living
room table, the gold and rust colored flower etchings on the glass
globes, the strong brass base, and the clear glass crystal chimney.

It's valuable. I know my antiques. I've studied them for years.
It's an authentic old-fashioned oil lamp, one like my grandmother
once had. I want it. I can't get that lamp out of my mind.

Brenda doesn't love it like I do. She lets it get dusty, and I
never see her use it, light the wick to softly brighten a room with a
beautiful glow. The lamp's not loved or cherished like it deserves
to be. My husband, Jack, doesn't love or cherish me anymore
either. I gained weight and lost my connection to the world when I
quit teaching to raise the two girls.

The lamp sits unused on Brenda's table next to her jade plants.
The plants. Several months ago, she asks me to water them while
she goes to Texas to look for a condo. "I'll be gone for at least

five weeks," she tells me. "I plan to retire soon and move there."

"Yes, I'd be glad to help you out," I say.

She hands me the key. "Madge, you don't know how much I appreciate this," she says. "I love all my plants, have babied them for years." I listen to her babble while I finger the key in my jean's pocket.

Brenda's been a good neighbor, a nurse. She doesn't work in a hospital though. She's one of those nurses who takes care of people in their own homes. She talks to me about my asthma, and she taught me how to use my inhaler. If I feel sick, she'll listen to my lungs and take my blood pressure. Once she asked me if I would like to attend a support group meeting for people with breathing problems. I told her I'm not interested.

She's always there if I need her, kind, friendly, and cheerful. I'm mad she's moving, leaving me behind. I seldom get to go on trips, have any fun. She's using me, only paying me a hundred dollars to water her plants for all those weeks. She thinks I have nothing better to do with my time now that the girls are in college.

I can't wait until she leaves so I can study the lamp up close without her around. When the day finally comes, I watch her back her car out of her garage. I peek behind my curtains to make sure she doesn't return for something she forgot. Her back seat is filled with suitcases and cardboard boxes. A half-hour later, I realize she's truly gone.

I grab her key and run out my door and across her yard. My hands tremble as I unlock her door and go inside. I rush toward the lamp. I caress it and run my fingers over the glass etchings.

Her phone rings. It startles me. I realize I can't keep standing there. I get up to leave. As I lock her door on the way out, I think about my grand- mother and how much she loved me. I miss her even though she's been dead for twenty years now.

After the first two days, I fall into a routine. Unless Jack is late leaving for work, I check on the lamp every morning about ten, after I've had my morning coffee. First, I turn it from side to side so I can see it from all different angles. I polish the glass globes until they sparkle from the sunlight that shines through the window. I daydream how beautiful the lamp will look in my house sitting on my hall table.

I must have the lamp. It belongs in my home with my other antiques, not in her house sitting on an old table by a stupid plant. She already has packed many of her things to take to her new house. She won't miss it. The day before she is scheduled to return home, she calls me. "Madge, I'll be here a little longer than I thought. I've called a realtor to put the house on the market. Could you water the plants a little longer?"

I hold back a sniffle. This could be bad news. Realtors will be in. I can't count on an empty house.

A week later a 'For Sale' sign sit in front of her house. Realtors and their clients come in and out of her place. I can't go and sit by the lamp anymore, but I think about it all the time.

I decide to take the lamp late at night when the neighbors are asleep. I'll put it in a box just in case anyone is spying on me. I must be careful not to fall or drop the box, but I can't carry a flashlight or candle to light my way, or someone may notice. It's a short distance between her house and mine, so I should be all right.

When I sleep, I dream about her and the lamp. In one dream I drop it; it crashes to the floor, breaking into thousands of picces.

I must get the lamp now, tonight. Otherwise, I will never rest.

I look out the window. The sky is dark, the stars and moon covered by the clouds. The night is warm but humid. A perfect night for a robbery. Funny how I know I'm stealing and some would call me a thief, but I think of myself as a rescuer, a do-it-yourself Martha Stewart.

It is just past midnight. Jack is sleeping in the guest room; he often sleeps there so his snoring doesn't awaken me. I go to the basement for an empty cardboard box and quietly let myself out my door. Sneaking across the yards, I tiptoe up Brenda's front steps and push her key into the lock and turn it until it clicks. A burning sensation starts in my stomach and rises to my throat. My hands shake. I open the door quickly and slip inside. I hear myself breathing fast. My legs are weak, and I plop down on her soft carpet. Her house is dark, but the moon shining through the windows illuminates the room and casts unusual shadows. It feels eerie. My heart pounds.

Can I pull this off? When I stand up and start walking, the floorboards squeak. I jump. What if she comes home unexpectedly? What will I say? Get a grip, I tell myself. Move fast and get out of here.

My trembling hands lower the lamp to the floor close to where I sit. What if I drop the lamp and it smashes just like in my dream? My lamp! I could lose it forever. I must control myself. I take deep breaths. My heart- beat slows. My hands become more steady.

I kiss the lamp gently. "You're mine now," I tell it. "I will take better care of you than her, love you more. My hall table will showcase you, so people can see you, enjoy you."

As I carefully slide the lamp into the box, I sense my grandmother's presence. When she was alive, we went to antique stores together. The ballerina doll with the painted face and black dancing shoes that she bought me for my seventh birthday has been lost for years. Grandma would hate that I'm stealing, but she'd understand. Like me, she knows the importance of being surrounded by beauty. I wish she were here tonight.

I cry softly as images of her playing dolls with me float through my mind. I carefully set the box on the steps outside Brenda's door, tears running down my cheeks. I close the door quietly and squint to locate the keyhole to lock the house back up. I lift the cardboard box and hug it to my chest.

Thinking of Grandma comforts me as I slink across the yard back to my house. I see car headlights down the street. Is it Brenda? I rush toward my porch, hoping to reach it before the car passes and the driver spots me. My foot catches on a tree root, I almost trip. No longer crying, I regain my balance. The lamp moves inside the box. Did it break? God, what am I doing? I want the lamp. I need it. I set the box down in the grass. The car whizzes by, the driver doesn't turn his head. I'm safe. The man didn't notice me. I open my front door, grab the box, and put it in the corner of my hall closet. I cover the box with an old coat, so Jack won't see it.

My forehead drips with sweat. I can't stand this anymore. I have to go to bed, forget about the lamp for a while, get some rest, find peace. I walk around my house feeling like someone else is in my body. Soon I'm in my bedroom. I drop down onto my comforter, hug my pillow, and fall asleep with wet tears on my cheeks.

I wake up the next morning with thoughts of lighting the lamp, but I need special oil. Why didn't I think of buying it earlier? No problem. I've been to *The Lamplifters Candle Shoppe* enough times to know their products.

When I get to the store, I test the aromas of the various oils and choose a soft pink vanilla-scented one. I'm going to use the lamp, not leave it to sit like a forgotten vacation souvenir. I rush back home eager to try out my purchases. When I take the lamp out of the box, I feel the blood rush to my face. My fingers tremble as I fill the glass base with oil, light a match, and hold it over the wick. Soon the lamp radiates a soft pink hue that outlines the golden flowers etched on the globe. I gasp at the beauty of it.

My throat chokes up so that I can hardly catch my breath.

I begin my days now by lighting the lamp and sitting in my

rocking chair staring at it. I sense Grandma's spirit by my side.

Three weeks later, the phone rings right before I am ready to go to bed. It's my neighbor. "I'm home," Brenda says. "I know it's late, but thanks for watering the plants. They look great. My oil lamp is missing though. I thought my son might have taken it, but he says no. Have you seen it?"

Oh, God. I have to keep my wits about me. I take a deep breath. "I don't remember seeing it. Maybe you packed it away before you left."

"No," Madge says. "I'm positive I didn't pack it. I loved that lamp. It's an old family heirloom. I have to find it. Tomorrow I'll file a police report to check if someone broke in, get fingerprints and all."

I break out in a cold sweat. What am I going to do? I didn't mean to be a thief. It didn't seem like I was stealing, just borrowing the lamp to take good care of it. I put the lamp back in its box and shoved it under the basement steps. Maybe she'll give up trying to find it and I can keep it and relax.

I lie down in bed and attempt to sleep. I toss. I turn. I wake up screaming trying to escape a policeman chasing me down an alley.

At dawn a peaceful dream enfolds me. It's Grandma hugging me. "Take the lamp back," she says. 'How?' I sense myself asking. Her vision fades, and I'm left with a sick feeling in the pit of my stomach and a splitting headache.

The wick is charred now. I rip it from the lamp and flush it down the toilet. Brenda will never notice it's missing. I carry the lamp globes to my bathtub and gently rinse the soot from them. I dry them carefully with my thickest bath towel and polish them until they shine.

I concoct a story and knock on her door. "Someone left your lamp on my porch," I tell her. "When I opened my door this morning to get the newspaper, there it sat. I can't believe it."

I feel her hesitate. Will she believe me? Will she yell, call the police, and ask me questions? My heart races. I am shaking so hard I have to lean against the door.

Brenda smiles. "Oh, thank you, Madge. How lucky. I was just on my way to the police station to report the theft. You made my day. Who left it at your house, do you think?"

"Probably a realtor or one of the buyers. They're in and out of houses all the time, know valuable things." My voice squeaks, and I feel a rattle in my throat.

She hugs me.

I'm off the hook. I've pulled it off. I'll never steal anything again. I'm no klepto. My muscles relax, and my trembling stops. I smile.

I walk back home and sit down in my rocking chair. The shaking starts again. I pull a pint of *Absolut* from under the side of the seat cushion. I unscrew the cap and lift the bottle to my lips. The warm vodka trickles all the way to the pit of my stomach.

I stand up slowly and lift her *Dresden* doll from the corner of my china closet. I run my fingers over the figurine's lace gown and her beautiful face and hair. Then, I take the doll by her ballerina slippers and fling it into my fireplace where it smashes into a thousand pieces.

I loved that doll. If I can't have it, no one else will.

THE GIFT EXCHANGE

The best place to succeed is where you are with what you have.
Charles M. Schwab

Kay Fletcher, a retired health department nurse, watched a woman about her own age work her way down the aisle toward the restrooms at the center of the plane. They would be landing in half an hour, and people were becoming restless after the long flight from Los Angeles to Washington, D.C. It struck her as rather sad that the woman in the aisle wore an outfit similar to both hers and the woman sitting beside her.

Kay's seatmate, who had introduced herself as Ellen O'Connor, would be visiting her daughter for the holidays, just as Kay would be visiting her son and his family. She supposed the three women, all dressed in the same kind of clothes, were in the same position, widows with no other family to visit at Christmas. She knew the look, wash and wear slacks with turtleneck jerseys and loose fitting jackets, similar to uniforms, only the colors varied.

"It was nice talking to you, Ellen. Maybe I'll see you again sometime."

"Too bad you're only staying four days. We could have dinner some night. It gets old being with the family for a week. The grandchildren resent having to be quiet; the kids and their parents walk around on tiptoes and are careful what they say lest they upset Grandma. Why can't we just have our own little club and forget the families?"

Kay laughed. "I wouldn't go that far, but I do admit to not being overly fond of my daughter-in-law, Brooke. She's a college professor. She directs research studies and teaches finance and international business courses. I think she regards all humans as objects for clinical research."

"My son-in-law disappears into the den the moment I arrive and doesn't come out 'til I leave. I only hope he doesn't behave like that when I'm not around. I do get the honor of seeing him at mealtimes. The kids say they only eat together as a family when I'm there. I suppose I could consider that my contribution to my grandchildren's upbringing. Social skills."

"My grandsons are involved in so many activities, I can't keep up with who's doing which sport or playing what instrument from week to week! Remember when we were teenagers? Friday night football games and sock hops. I was a cheerleader for a while. And when I lived in a college dorm, the boys and girls stayed in separate buildings."

They agreed times had changed and promised to call each other when they got back to Los Angeles. Before getting off the plane, they exchanged e-mail addresses and phone numbers. When she entered the airport, Kay dropped Ellen's into the nearest trash can. Years of experience had taught her she'd never hear from the woman again.

Her son, Gary, met her at the baggage claim; and after a brief greeting, the two headed out to the parking lot for the short drive to the suburbs. "Brooke's invited a couple for dinner on Christmas. She wanted me to warn you so it wouldn't be too much of a shock."

Kay laughed. "How can company be a shock? I assume you

socialize and entertain from time to time. It'll be fun to meet some of your friends. Who are they?"

Gary, her tall athletic boy of forty-two, grinned. "You might not like it, Mom. Two Chinese refugees who don't speak English."

She raised her eyebrows at that. "Hmm. That should be interesting. Are they even Christians?"

"I don't know. But does it matter? Anyway, Brooke's teaching an international finance class at the college and learned about them from another professor. She thought it would be helpful to her research."

"You know I'm interested in different cultures. I can't imagine what they'll think of our Christmas." Kay nodded, acknowledging both her son's comments and her own opinion of Brooke's relationships. "We could end up sitting in silence and staring at each other over the turkey."

"I don't think it will be that grim, Mom. Come on, you're tired now; but you'll get into the spirit of things once you've had a shower and a rest."

"What I really want, my dear, is…"

"I know. I have a pitcher of martinis already made up for you. We'll have one the minute we get in the door. Brooke has hors d'oeuvres prepared, and then we'll be ready to sit around and talk. James and Scott will be home around ten. They went to a movie with friends."

Gary pulled into the driveway shortly before seven. Kay hurried into the house, unused to the bitter cold. She'd moved to Los Angeles over thirty years ago.

Brooke stood by the front door and turned her cheek for a kiss from Kay, which Kay dutifully presented, although she would have preferred a welcoming hug. "So glad you could make it,

Mother. Gary, take your mother's things to the guest room. I'll get the drinks. Unless, of course, you'd rather have a nap before dinner."

Kay looked at this cool woman, who was the love of her son's life. She was of medium height and weight and wore her short blonde hair drawn back from her face. She rarely put on any make-up, so Kay was pleased to see she'd made an effort, using pink lip gloss and blue eye shadow to enhance her startling blue eyes. The eyes, because of their thick dark lashes, were her best feature.

"The drinks and snacks will be perfect. I napped a bit on the flight."

"Did Gary warn you about the guests coming tomorrow?" Brooke asked as she headed toward the kitchen.

"Just that they don't speak English. It should make for an interesting visit."

Brooke opened the refrigerator and handed a tray of food to Kay. "You can unwrap these and put them on the coffee table."

"Tell me about these people," asked Kay.

"I don't know many details, only that they're middle aged. One's a retired chemical engineer and the other a pediatrician. I want to make the day perfect for them."

"At least they're well educated," Kay said with a laugh, hoping to make light of a situation Brooke seemed to regard as ripe for worry and stress. "I used to work with people from a variety of cultures when I was at the health department. I still do with my editing job. Perhaps, I'll be able to ease any tension that arises."

"You mustn't worry yourself, Mother. We can handle everything. The boys plan to sing Christmas carols. We'll show them our photo albums from some of our trips. I have everything timed down to the last minute."

Kay was relieved when her son returned and poured the drinks. They spent the evening hearing all about Brooke's international finance class. Kay wished Gary would have talked more about his work at the Art Museum. By the time the boys came in at ten-thirty, she was ready for bed even though her body was still on LA time.

The following day, Christmas arrived along with a raging snowstorm. Brooke worked in the kitchen, leaving Kay to watch the boys play new video games on the television, while Gary tried to stay ahead of the heavy snow rapidly accumulating in the driveway. By one o'clock, the boys had been included in the snow shoveling challenge to keep the driveway clear.

Inside, Brooke set the table with her finest linens and china, assuring Kay that she had no need of help. By two o'clock, Gary decided it would be safer to let a cab driver assume the risk of transporting the refugees from DC to the house and called for a taxi.

Two snow encrusted people entered the home at three-thirty. They were so heavily wrapped that Kay couldn't tell if they were men or women. She surprised her family by saying, "*Ni Hao,*" to the guests.

"*Ni Hao Ma,*" a masculine voice responded. Brooke hurried in to take their coats and sent them off to the laundry room with Gary. Then the introductions began. They each pointed to themselves, pronouncing their names several times until it seemed everyone understood. The two Chinese people turned out to be siblings named Wu, first names, Minsheng and Huiqing.

Through hand signals and much laughter, the Wu's made it clear they were brother and sister. Mr. Wu had lost a spouse during periods of civil unrest; but neither Kay, nor anyone else, could work out the details. Dr. Wu had never married. Brooke brought out her photo albums while the boys sat on cushions on the floor looking embarrassed for their mother; but the Wu's smiled, their heads bobbing as they looked at the pictures.

At five o'clock the power went off, which meant the lovely turkey dinner stopped cooking. Gary and the boys put together a fire in the fireplace. As they worked to bring in wood from the garage, Mr. Wu contributed to the effort by placing a piece of newspaper on top of the kindling and setting it alight. Since Gary had not yet opened the flue, smoke quickly filled the room, triggering the smoke alarms in the house. Mr. Wu moved out of the way, repeating "*Dui Bu Qi*" each time anyone looked at him. Kay explained that he was apologizing. Brooke opened the living room windows while the boys ran to the back of the house to open the sliding door for cross ventilation.

As the house aired, it cooled so rapidly Gary and Brooke had to find extra sweaters and blankets for everyone. The boys brought in flashlights and candles from the kitchen.

Kay chuckled to herself about her daughter-in-law's plight. The carefully scripted day no longer existed. Now they sat in glowing candlelight singing Christmas carols for a couple who hadn't a clue what the words meant. She watched Mr. Wu gallantly smile in appreciation of the family's efforts while his sister looked more and more miserable as time went by.

Scott, the fourteen year old, ran upstairs and returned with a *Game Boy* and showed it to Dr. Wu. Her eyes lit up at the sight of something familiar; and the two of them played happily for a while until Gary cleared his throat to gain everyone's attention. "I made some phone calls from my Smart phone. The power is on in some areas. I checked and found an Indian restaurant not too far away. I think we should all go there for dinner. What do you say?"

Brooke glared. "But the turkey…"

"It's probably poison by now. Half cooked. Sitting in the oven for hours. I'm afraid it'll have to go."

The boys shouted, "Hurrah." At the sound of their cheers, the

Wu's smiled and nodded. Kay added her assent. Brooke went for the coats.

Kay sat in the rear of the van with the Wu's. The rest of the family used the individual seats at the front of the vehicle. With hand signals and Kay's limited knowledge of some Chinese words, they carried on a conversation during the ride to the restaurant. By the time they arrived, the three of them acted like old pals.

"Mom," Gary asked once they were seated and had ordered drinks, "When did you learn Chinese?"

"I only know a few words. You know about my nursing work at the health department. And I've told you about my new job. I've learned a lot about different languages through the years."

"You said you were editing scripts."

"I work for a publisher. I'm their health editor. I read all kinds of stories but mainly edit for continuity. You know, to make sure the twenty-four year old blonde nurse in the first scene hasn't become inexplicably a forty-year-old brunette in the fifth scene. Or, if she started out as a Registered Nurse, isn't now a Licensed Practical Nurse. I quite enjoy my job. It's almost as transcultural as my health department work.

"That's cool, Grandma. Mom and Dad never told us what you do. Did you start that after Grandpa died?"

"James!" Brooke hastened to scold the boy. "Don't upset your grandmother."

"She's not upset. Are you, Grandma?" the boy asked.

"Do I look upset? I was extremely distressed when your grandfather died, but we had a good life together. He's the one who introduced me to the publisher. I feel as if he's with me every day I'm at my job."

It took several minutes of gesticulating and much nodding and bobbing of heads for Kay to catch the Wu's up to date on the conversation. By then, Mr. Wu had been able to explain that he preferred to be called Minsheng. She told him to call her Kay.

Minsheng used a paper napkin to draw a picture, which he handed to Kay. It was of a Chinese woman dressed in slacks with a loose fitting jacket over a high-necked shirt. He pointed to his drawing and then to Kay's outfit, which closely resembled the one she had worn on the plane. She gathered from his continued smiling and nodding that he approved.

While the others worked to decipher the Indian restaurant's menu, Kay and Minsheng worked to decipher each other's drawings on the rapidly diminishing supply of paper napkins.

By the time their *Mulligatawny* soup arrived, the waiter had replaced the napkins with a notepad. Huiqing continued to play with the *Game Boy* throughout dinner, happily sharing her skill strategies with Scott.

At the end of the evening when they put the Wu's in a taxi in front of the restaurant, Minsheng handed Kay his e-mail address. She tucked it in her wallet behind her driver's license.

CHANGE OF HEART

Faced with a crisis, the man of character falls back onto himself.
Charles DeGaulle

Frank, my Frank, my handsome husband, where have you gone? Your dementia has taken over our lives and left me feeling as if I'm all alone, stranded on a faraway island. Your wavy black hair that I once finger combed for hours now hangs drably over your ears. It's turned a dull gray, dark in the back with silver strands at your temples. Some days it's oily, some days not, depending on whether or not you let me shampoo it. And your legs, once firm and muscular are now heavy, hairless and flabby; your feet sometimes are swollen around the ankles. You wear white cotton socks and canvas tennis shoes for safe walking these days. Our lives have taken a 180-degree turn from five years ago. I've become your caregiver.

* * *

In the early years, Frank was always there for me day and night. It seemed like only yesterday that we would argue politics, go to the shore with the kids, play eighteen holes of golf, and listen to classical music sipping Merlot in our king-sized bed. And sing. Frank loved to sing. For a while he sang with jazz bands in Chicago's Old Town bars and restaurants. The patrons cheered his smile, lively stage movements, and deep baritone voice. "We want Frank," they shouted to the club manager. Those days are over.

* * *

The changes began over two years ago-his reckless driving, his impatience with waitresses in restaurants, his disinterest in showering and bathing, his problems with his co-workers at the engineering firm where he worked. Finally, I called our family physician, who referred Frank to Dr. Lewis, a geriatrician specializing in the diagnosis and treatment of dementia. After the battery of tests and the examination, we sat in his office on straight backed wooden chairs waiting to hear the diagnosis.

He looked at us kindly, a gentle smile on his face. "The memory, impulsive behavior, and faltering speech problems are probably Alzheimer's."

I looked over at Frank, who was staring straight ahead, his eyes fixed on the black pen in the doctor's white lab coat. Tears welled up in the corner of his eyes. He started to speak but then choked back a sob.

"Frank's only fifty-seven," I said.

Dr. Lewis ran his fingers over his balding head. "Carol, I know he's young, but these behaviors aren't limited to seventy and eighty year olds."

I shook my head in disbelief. "We've been married for thirty-two years. He's rarely been sick."

"We did a complete study. There are medications. Things might even out for a long time."

We walked from the office in a daze. When we got home, we lay next to each other in bed each other's arms while we cried and talked about our future. "It's not fair. I'm too young. We're finally alone, empty nesters. We had so many plans and now this."

I ran my fingers through his thinning hair. "We'll get through this, Frank. There are medications, experimental treatments. We'll find an answer."

He jerked his head away. "Thank God, Sandra is married and has Nelson. I don't want her to feel obligated to take care of me. She has her own life now."

I put my arms around him. "I'll always be there for you. I'll be the one to manage things, not our daughter. I'm strong. I won't weaken. You'll be with me. We'll stay together, nothing will break us apart."

"You'll get tired, Carol, just like Mom did with Dad. She never left him, but she wanted to a lot of times in those eleven years it took for Alzheimer's Disease to kill him. You might leave me, find another man."

"I'll never leave you for anything or anyone." I crossed my heart to make the words even stronger. "You'll always be the love of my life." I held him tightly until he became quiet.

* * *

From that day on, we wrapped our arms around each other before we fell asleep. Sometimes, I woke up in the middle of the night in a cold sweat, my heart racing. I couldn't imagine what I would do if I no longer could take care of him. He was my sweetheart. I'd known him since we were sophomores in high school. He would never go to a nursing home. Tears filled my eyes, and I wanted to pound my pillow, but I stayed completely still, so I didn't wake Frank.

Over the next two years, Frank's condition deteriorated. The day he took the car out and didn't come home for two hours because he got lost in the neighborhood, I hid his car keys. The afternoon he wandered off when I was napping, I called a handyman to install an alarm on the front door. He often got out of bed at night and paced back and forth, organizing and rearranging his clothes in his closets and drawers and his tools in the basement. His roller-coaster emotions ranged from moments of mild and mellow behavior with periods of screaming and swearing. Evenings were the worst; right before dark Frank was the most fragile. I talked to him in a flat but warm voice not letting excitement or anger into my speech; he'd become extremely sensitive to any stimulation. I had learned to predict his behavior and manage it with music and anti-depressants. When he was singing or dancing with me, he acted almost normal; so I manipulated his activities by waltzing him around.

My body wasn't cooperating. Pain shot through my lower back when I bathed him. I lost over twenty pounds. When I looked in the mirror, an old woman with gray hair, a gaunt face, and stooped shoulders stared back at me. Even though I was only fifty-nine, I felt exhausted most of the time. Driving home from the grocery store last Friday, I fell asleep at a red light, shocked to be awakened by honking horns.

I was at my wit's end. I felt proud to have honored my commitment to keep Frank safe and comfortable, but his dementia was driving me crazy. I began to stare at handsome men in the grocery store or the bank and undress them with my eyes, longing for a sensitive man's touch, someone to hold me like Frank used to do. When I came home and looked at my husband, I wondered how I could be so self-centered. Emotionally I was no longer by his side. Anger filled my heart, anger that I no longer led a normal life.

* * *

I called the Alzheimer's Association and talked to a nurse, Deanna Clancy. She assured me that my feelings were normal and invited me to a support group for caregivers where I met other spouses like me. Deanna constantly told me that I must take care of myself, find something pleasurable to do every day. "Even getting a job a day or two a week may be helpful," she said. "I can give you information on a reputable agency that specializes in home health aides for dementia patients."

The following week I hired an aide, Janice, who stayed with

Frank for a few hours every week while I did my grocery shopping and ran errands. When I accepted a part-time job teaching English Literature at the local community college, Janice agreed to work extra hours.

* * *

I first met Vincent at my nephew's wedding reception over a year ago. It was my only outing in weeks, and I had tinted my hair with highlights to match the gold in my evening dress. He sat next to me at small round table in the back corner of the room. His hazel green eyes and light complexion were so different from Frank's. Vincent and I sipped champagne and talked about recent books we had read. I learned he was a teacher, an English major like me, who worked at the high school, not far from where I taught at the community college.

When there was a pause in the conversation, he said, "Will you dance with me, Carol?"

I felt myself blush. "I'm married, you know. My husband, Frank, is at home with a nurse's aide. He has Alzheimer's. I miss him terribly tonight. This is one of the few times I've been out without him since he got sick."

"I understand, but dance with me anyway. It's only a dance. I was married for twenty years but have been divorced for the last three."

Vincent took my hand and gently led me to the dance floor. I hadn't danced for years, but I remembered the two-step, and soon we were whirling around the room along with the other couples.

His hand lightly brushed my breast. My attraction to him surprised me.

"Can I call you sometimes, just as a friend?" he asked as we left the reception hall.

I paused. "Just as a friend."

He phoned me two weeks after the wedding, asking me to lunch to critique a short story he had written.

Surprised yet flattered, I agreed to meet him for coffee at *Starbuck's*. We talked for an hour about his writing aspirations.

"I love to write about beautiful women, women who look like you, Carol."

"Thank you." My heart skipped a beat. I balled up the paper napkin in my hand.

"My treat next week," he said. *"Ruby Tuesday's* at three, right after school."

I surprised myself by saying yes. Soon my calendar had Vincent penciled in every Thursday from three to five. I couldn't believe how easily I drew him into my life and how much I wanted him to stay.

Vincent. I would never have appreciated him several years ago. His professional demeanor, his quiet reflections, his short curly blond hair, his designer suits and leather briefcase. His soft smile and gentle hands, the way he caressed my arm when I was upset. His strong, assertive personality. His quick mind helped me think through my dilemmas, and his compassionate spirit lightened my heart. His body stimulated me, excited me, and comforted me in a way I'd never known with Frank. I felt young again.

"You need to get out, take care of yourself, have some fun. Not stay home every evening taking care of Frank. Let yourself go," he told me.

It frustrated me that I couldn't see Vincent more often. Getting a sitter for evenings was difficult. Frank hated it when I left him after dark and clung to me when I started to go out the door.

"I'm afraid," He often mumbled. His face haunted me when we were apart, yet I constantly planned ways to get out of the house, get away from him.

Frank and Vincent. I saw myself with both these men and compared them to each other. I played one against the other in my mind. I no longer trusted the woman I had become.

Saturday night. Vincent's birthday. I made secret plans for our daughter and her husband to watch Frank. I told Sandra and Nelson I was going to a work-related wine tasting party and would return late.

"We'll take Dad out for dinner. Don't worry, Mom," Sandra told me.

"Eating with Dad in a restaurant could be difficult." I said. "Be prepared for anything."

* * *

After Vincent and I finished our dinners, we were still in a festive mood. "Let's drop in at the jazz club over on Tenth Street for some music and dancing before we head back to my place," he suggested.

I hesitated. Frank and I used to go to that club. Finally I agreed. "Okay, just for a little bit. We don't have much time. Someday, darling, I will spend the whole night with you." I kissed his cheek.

"You feel guilty being with me. I don't care that you're married; you're married in name only. Your marriage ended when Frank got sick."

"The marriage vows didn't say that, Vincent; but you're right, I feel guilty being with you, yet I'm with you anyway."

When we walked through the door of *The Tribute*, I thought I heard Frank's voice. God. Was I crazy? No, there he was, Frank, my Frank, on stage singing 'Let me Call You Sweetheart,' smiling and swaying to the piano player's music. Frank, my beloved husband; he looked handsome again. His hair was parted on the side and neatly combed away from his face. Simple khakis and a long sleeved blue button-down shirt made him look young, hid his illness somehow. A glow radiated from his eyes, a glow I hadn't

140

seen for months. His singing was off key, some words were wrong, but I was amazed he remembered them at all. Sandra and Nelson, both nodding their heads to the rhythm, sat at a center table, directly in front of Frank. I recognized the group on stage as cronies of Frank's from the old days.

I stood at the doorway for an instant longer. My heart pounded in my chest. Tears filled my eyes. "We have to go. It's Frank. He's in there. On stage. I can't see you anymore." I rushed out into the parking lot. Vincent ran after me.

"Carol, wait, wait," he yelled from the curb. He caught up to me and took my arm.

"I can't," I whispered. "I have to leave. Take me home."

Vincent hesitated. He turned me to face him; I ran my fingers across his cheek. "Carol, I love you." His voice cracked, and he kissed me gently at the side of my eye where a tear had formed.

I looked into his hazel eyes and saw caring there. "I love you, too, Vincent. You've made me feel like a woman again." I pulled away and put my hand on his cheek. "Good-bye and thank you."

He hugged me gently. "I'm here for you, Carol, if you change your mind."

"Please go home. And don't call me anymore. I'm not ready to leave the club yet. I'll call a taxi later."

He stroked my hair, then turned away and stepped into his Grand Prix. I watched his car slowly go down the street. Then, I walked back into the restaurant and sat at an empty table in the back of the club. I ordered a diet soda and sipped it while I shredded a paper napkin into small pieces. Tears filled my eyes.

Frank, my beloved Frank. How could I have ever forsaken you?

THE POTTER'S WHEEL

Commitment is an act, not a word.

Jean-Paul Sartre

Matthew downs another shot of tequila and is rewarded by a kiss from Susan, who's sitting on his lap. Two kisses for three shots. He contemplates a fourth. It's his twenty-first birthday, and his Phi Delt brothers at Syracuse University have organized a party in the fraternity house. Just as he lifts his glass, his smart phone rings.

Matthew unravels himself from Susan and sets down his glass to pull his phone from his pocket. With unsteady feet he lifts himself from the brown tweed sofa and walks to the corner of the room. "Quiet, guys. Shut up for a minute so I can hear."

He touches the phone's screen expecting to hear his family singing "Happy Birthday" like they did last year. Instead it's his mother and she sounds serious. "It's Denise, Matthew. She's taken a bad turn. She needs a new kidney. Can you come home tonight? Doctor Lyon wants to meet with us all tomorrow." His mother's voice cracks. "I'm sorry, Matthew. I know it's your birthday, but…"

"Mom, can't it wait 'til Thursday?"

"We don't have time to spare. Come tonight. It'll take you three hours to get here. We need to be in his office at nine in the morning."

Matthew takes a deep breath. "God, why didn't you tell me sooner? The guys are having a party for me."

"I hear them, Matthew. Please come."

He remembers how Denise played catch with him in the backyard when he was a Little League pitcher and how she shared her Halloween candy with him and not their brother, Alex. She even did his high school algebra homework. "I'll be there, Mom."

Matthew slowly disconnects. "It was my mom. My sister's real sick. The party'll have to wait. I gotta go home." He stumbles back to his chair. Susan sits on a footstool in front of him.

She squeezes his knee and runs her fingers over his muscular shoulders. "You can't drive like that, Matt. You've had too much to drink."

Matthew looks at the frat wall covered with framed photos of every graduation class since 1942. Taking a deep breath, he wonders what problems all those guys had to deal with on their twenty-first birthday. Shaking his head, he says. "I'll get some food in me. In a couple of hours, I'll be okay."

"I'll make you scrambled eggs and coffee. Then you can take off." She runs her fingers through his curly blonde hair.

He takes a deep breath. "Uh…thanks, Susan. Good idea. I'll get my things packed and leave in a couple of hours. Mom wants me to move back home 'til this is over; it may be awhile until we can see each other."

She pulls his face to hers and rubs her lips against his. "God, Matt. I'll miss you."

* * *

The next day Matthew sits with his family in Dr. Lyon's office.

The doctor looks directly at him. "Denise needs a kidney transplant. Any family member is good, but a sibling is usually a better match. Maybe one of you two brothers. If you can both stay a few minutes, we'll do blood testing and tissue typing."

"All right," Matthew mumbles, praying he won't be a match. He turns his head away from the doctor's probing eyes, clenching his fists until his nails push into the palms of his hands.

Dr. Lyon nods. "The lab is down the hall."

As they walk to the lab, Matthew playfully cuffs his older brother, Alex, on the shoulder. "I wonder which one of us it will be. If we're both a match, we can flip a coin."

As they wait for the technician to draw their blood, Alex forces a laugh. "I'm betting on you." He looks at his watch. "Hope this is fast. I gotta get back to work."

The lab work goes smoothly. "We'll have the results to Dr. Lyon tomorrow," she tells them.

Alex rushes out the door before Matthew has a chance to say goodbye.

* * *

The phone call at his parent's house comes two days later. "Matthew, it's Katie with Dr. Lyon. You're the best match. Alex is our second choice."

Matthew gulps. "I'm not sure I can do it."

"I understand. It can be frightening. The nurse on the transplant team would be a good person to talk with. I can fit you in her schedule tomorrow."

"Not tomorrow. Maybe Monday. I'll call."

"Don't wait longer than that. We don't have much time."

"I said I'd call." His voice sounds louder than he intends.

Matthew grabs his jacket from the hall closet and jumps in his car. At first, he drives aimlessly around the city, tears running down his cheeks. Die! Denise dead. He can't imagine it. His grandpa died when he was old and walked with a cane. Denise. She's only twenty-nine.

At sunset, he's driving along curvy mountain roads in the Catskills where Uncle Ian lives. Perhaps, that's where he had intended to go all along.

* * *

Uncle Ian lives in an apartment above his pottery studio, which takes up the entire first floor of an eighty-year-old wooden frame house sheltered by overgrown birch and evergreen trees. Several discolored pottery wheels are lined up against one wall. A kiln sits in the corner of the other. Scraps of broken clay, some painted and some not, lay on the dusty floor. Year after year, the studio remains unchanged; today the sameness comforts Matthew. He takes a deep breath to compose himself before he enters the shop. The cool air permeating the room and the earthy smell, like damp garden dirt after a summer rain, refresh him.

Ian's shoulder length hair, once a vibrant brown, is now duller, grayer, and thinner and his beard is scraggly. Yet even at fifty-nine, he's maintained his athletic build and added a new heart-shaped tattoo to his muscular right hand. Only the color and plaid of his flannel shirts have changed over the years. Faded denim overalls, usually covered with wet clay and frayed at the knees, are a constant.

Ian served as a medic in the Viet Nam War. After he came home, he had terrible nightmares of the bloody suffering he had seen. Since then, he's become quiet, rarely talking about himself or the war; Uncle Ian is the best listener Matthew knows. Some consider him a recluse, he's lived alone so long; but Matthew has always admired his simple life style. He remembers their late night talks about girls, drinking, and ways to deal with bullies and that it was Uncle Ian who stayed in the hospital overnight with him after he had his appendix out on his twelfth birthday.

His uncle looks up from the clay he is kneading. "Hey, Matt. It's good to see you. What brings you here this time of day? Classes over?"

"I came home for Denise. Since she's sick, the Profs are letting me finish my classes with independent studies. I'll have my business degree next month."

"Good for you. Your dad told me about Denise. Wish her I could give her a kidney. I went to be tested at the VA, but I'm not a match. What going on with you?" He motions for Matthew to sit across the table from him.

"I'm a mess," he blurts out. "They want my kidney."

Ian throws the ball of clay on his wheel. "Hmm." He squeezes the clay between his fingers.

"The doctor says I'm the best match. Denise… Denise is dying. I care but maybe not enough. I don't want to go under the knife. I might die. I want her to live more than anything. But without me losing my kidney." Tears come to his eyes. "I stayed awake all night. Every time I closed my eyes, I saw her face."

Ian wipes his hands on a towel and pats him on the shoulder. "I prayed it would never come to this."

"Uncle Ian, you were a medic. What do you know about kidneys? Can a person really live with only one? Would it make that much difference to Denise?"

Ian stops working the clay and leans back. Matt thinks he might tumble backward off his stool, but Ian raises a knee and wraps his arms around it. He frowns for a moment before speaking. "First, Matt, sure. People can live with one kidney. Ever since Denise got sick, I've been reading about transplants. I never went to medical school. Got drafted for the war when I was nineteen before I had a chance to make up my mind about college. One thing I know for sure, Matt, is the doctors will do everything they can for both of you and it's the most normal thing in the world to be scared."

"They want to do a lot of tests on me."

"The docs want to make sure you're healthy, that it won't hurt you to have only one kidney. Blood tests, heart and lung checks, and a kidney X- ray using dye."

Matthew frowns. "That's a lot to go through."

Ian nods. "And they'll want you to see a psychiatrist to make sure you can cope with the stress of the surgery and that nobody is forcing you to have the operation."

"A shrink. What if he thinks I'm nuts?"

Ian laughs. "I know better. Let him talk to me." He takes another wad of clay and rolls it into a ball.

Matthew kicks a piece of hardened clay lying by his foot. "Will my kidney work in Denise?"

"There are no guarantees, but it's the best chance she has. Rejection is always possible. Take a few days. Think about it."

"Doesn't feel like I have much choice. Mom and Dad would both hate me if I said no. They love Denise most. She's the only girl."

"You know they love you, too. Imagine having children and this kind of problem. What would you do? Remember your Bible stories? Solomon cutting the baby in half? Well, this is kind of like that, isn't it? They're asking you to cut only a little bit from yourself to give to your sister. Did they say you had to do it?"

"I can't talk to them about it. Mom cries, and Dad stares out into space. It's like he's not even there."

"Take this clay, and roll it while you talk. Molding clay helps me make sense out of life."

Reluctantly, Matthew picks up the gray clay, moister than the first batch, and sticks his fingers into it. The feeling of the mushy clay between his fingers reminds him of playing in the mud when he was young. His muscles relax.

"Since Denise has been sick, going on four years now, the household revolves around her. Is she watching her salt and fluid intake? Is she getting enough rest? Is she going out with her friends? Mom's calendar has Denise written on it for almost every day of the week. And driving her to dialysis and doctor appointments. We all take turns. I'm tired of it all. The second I get home for Christmas or spring break, my time's spent relieving Mom and Dad of the constant driving. I feel like a servant, not a son. I know they love me, but it's like I'm a non-person, a robot."

"You've been a good brother."

"Now they're asking me to miss my graduation, the parties, and the celebration of my work these past four years. And, Uncle Ian, this is probably the hardest to admit, but it's an operation! It'll hurt. If I don't do it, they'll all hate me and think I'm a baby." He throws the ball of clay on the floor and wipes his nose on his sweatshirt sleeve.

Uncle Ian finally speaks. "They want what's best for all of you. Most parents would be devastated to see their child as sick as Denise." He hands Matthew another ball of clay. "Use this old wheel of mine. Throw this piece of clay on it, roll it, and see what happens."

For several minutes, Matthew squeezes the ball of clay in his hands. Then he slams it on the wheel and starts to spin it. "Alex should be the match. He's five years older."

"You and Alex never seemed that close. How come?"

"I wish we got along better. I've always looked up to him. He thinks Mom spoils me. Two years ago we had a big fight when he left my motorcycle outside overnight and someone stole it. And when I wrecked his car, he didn't speak to me for weeks. Now he thinks he's cool because he makes a lot of money selling

148

computer software and has set a date to get married in May."

"I can understand your feelings. I was never that close to your dad, who's six years younger than me. We get along well now though, although we both have a loner streak, me more so. Time is a healer."

"Would you give Dad one of your kidneys?"

Ian scratches his chin. "I suppose I might. But you don't have to have the operation, Matthew. You don't have to do it." Ian pauses. "It's a chance though to give, give something no one else can, to save your sister's life. How would you feel later if she died and you had said no?"

"I dunno."

"Ever thought you might feel guilty if you didn't?"

Matthew takes a deep breath. "Yeah, I would feel real guilty. I want Denise to live. She's my sister and more important than my kidney. I know that I can live with just one kidney, for now anyway. But what if something happens to the other one? The doctor warned me not to play football or con- tact sports so I don't injure it. Maybe these kidney infections are a family thing."

"See this extra pottery wheel of mine? It's yours to use. Come to the studio anytime. You're artistic. Get some clay and mold it while you think about what you want to do. Stay the week-end, 'til Monday."

"All right. I'll call Mom and let her know."

The next morning, Matthew gets up early to make breakfast for Uncle Ian—pancakes, hash browns, sausage patties with biscuits, orange juice and coffee. They eat sitting at Ian's picnic table under the evergreen tree where squirrels are busy finding acorns and scurrying away with them.

"You've helped me a lot, Uncle Ian. I'll do it, give Denise my kidney. Something about squishing clay through my fingers helped me think straight. I just hope the kidney works."

"You do your part. The rest is out of your control."

"It's been good being here. Thanks." Matthew hugs Ian good-bye before he gets in the car to head back home.

* * *

The next afternoon, he visits Denise in the hospital. Not having eaten all day, his head is throbbing as he walks into her room. He sits down on a wooden chair by the side of her bed.

Goosebumps cover his arms and legs when he sees how pale and thin she has become. Her brown curly hair is dull and brittle, and her ankles sticking out from under her blanket are puffy. As he takes her dry hand in his and feels her bony fingers, a lump forms in his throat. Memories of the summer they spent weeks building a tree house in the woods behind their house swirl through his mind.

He leans forward and looks into her hazel green eyes. "I'm the one. Out of all of us, I'm the best match."

She pushes the control button to raise the head of her hospital bed. "I don't want you to lose your kidney, Matt. You're too young. I thought Alex would be the match."

"Nope, as I said, I'm the one. The best of the four of us." He runs his fingers across her cheek.

"Are you sure?" Denise whispers, picking at a patch of loose threads from her spread.

"Hey, it'll be easier on me than you," he lies. "You'd better take good care of my kidney." He laughs a little too loudly.

She sighs, then brushes her hand over his face and runs her fingers through his hair. Looking into his dark blue eyes, she says, "My kid brother. I don't know why this is happening, why I'm so sick. I'm sorry, but I love you and owe you big time."

Matthew swallows hard. He can't believe what he just said.

150

* * *

The surgery is scheduled for the following Tuesday. When Matthew arrives at the hospital with his parents, he sees Uncle Ian waiting for them by the information desk and breathes a sigh of relief.

"Where's Alex?" he asks.

Uncle Ian frowns. "I don't know about Alex but this is my third time out of the mountains in five years. Made you a good luck charm."

Ian hands him a handmade amulet shaped like a potter's wheel with Matthew's name etched in Egyptian hieroglyphics. "They won't let you take it to the operating room, but it'll be here for you when you wake up."

In the surgical area, Matthew signs the consent form. His hand shakes as he writes his name, but his signature is firm and clear.

Wearing a hospital gown and plastic armband, he's wheeled into the preoperative holding area. His parents and Uncle Ian lean over and hug him.

"We love you. We'll be here all day," his mom says. Her blue eyes linger over him longer than usual.

Ian's lightly punches Matthew in the chest. "I'm proud of you, Matt." Matthew shrugs and gives Ian a high-five.

"But where's Alex?" His mother glances at his dad. "He must have been called into work."

Soon Matthew is wheeled into the pre-operative holding area. "Make it fast," he tells the nurse. "Put me out. I can't think about this anymore." He focuses on rolling an imaginary ball of clay in his hands until the needle hits his vein.

* * *

When Matthew wakes up after the surgery, Uncle Ian is sitting beside his bed.

"The operation's over, Matt. Your mom and dad have been back and forth between you and Denise all day. They just left. They're exhausted."

Ian spoon feeds Matthew ice chips and keeps a cool washcloth on his forehead.

Matthew spots the amulet on his bedside stand and reaches for it. He runs his fingers over the etching and lifts his hands up and tries to put the amulet around his neck. Uncle Ian helps him.

"I'm not taking this off for a long time, Uncle Ian."

Both surgeries are successful. Denise's condition improves dramatically as her new kidney begins to function. Uncle Ian and his parents visit every day. Alex comes in once.

"Sorry I haven't been here more. It's the boss. He has me working sixty hours a week. And the wife has a long to-do list for me on the week-ends."

Matthew shrugs. "Whatever, no big deal."

* * *

Matthew misses his college graduation and the festivities that went along with it, but he no longer cares about that or that Susan has broken up with him. He's grateful for the successful surgeries, his business administration degree and the financial analyst job in the city waiting for him.

After he recuperates at his parent's home, he moves to a rented townhouse in the city. At first, he's excited; but, months later, finds his financial analyst job and being stuck in a third floor office high-rise with thirty other employees frustrating. He begins his work week with a heavy heart waiting for the weekends when he can drive up to Uncle Ian's studio.

Matthew uses Ian's potter's wheel to create plates, bowls, and pots for his uncle to display at local art fairs. People like his pottery, and many of his pieces are sold. To Matthew's surprise,

Ian pays him for his work. He thinks about leaving his corporate job and becoming an artist like Uncle Ian but it scares him too much to give up the money and security the job offers.

* * *

Denise's body accepts the new kidney, and she returns to her first grade teaching position. Color returns to her face, and the puffiness around her ankles disappears. She enrolls in a Wednesday night Yoga class and signs up to be a Yoga instructor. "I'm happier than I've been in months," she tells Matthew.

A year later, Denise complains of being tired. "Rejection," Dr. Lyon says. "I'm sorry. We'll try dialysis again."

She can no longer work and is granted medical disability. For a few weeks, her health improves with more dialysis, medications, and rest. Months later her kidney shuts down again, and she moves back home with her parents. As Denise becomes weaker, a hospital bed is set up in the den. Dr. Lyon predicts she has fewer than six months to live and makes a referral to hospice.

* * *

Matthew moves back into his old bedroom and takes several weeks of unpaid time off work to help care for his sister. He seldom has time to go to Uncle Ian's and use the potter's wheel.

A hospice nurse, Heidi, visits the family every Monday and Thursday. She adjusts Denise's medications and teaches the family how to care for her.

"Call me anytime, day or night," she tells them.

One day Matthew is talking to Heidi in the living room. He's sprawled on the sofa; she's sitting across from him on a recliner chair.

He runs his hands through his hair. "Most evenings, I read Denise several pages of *The Hobbitt*, her favorite book now, until she falls asleep. I even learned to paint her fingernails the 'ice and fire' red that she likes. I bring her fresh daisies every day. They're her favorite flower."

Heidi leans toward him and takes his hand in hers. "I wish all my patients had someone like you. You're very caring, but I know how hard these eight weeks have been for you."

"I've gotten afraid to live my life without her. I don't know how I'll manage. Who will I give water to drink through a straw? Whose hair will I brush? Whose tears will I wipe away?"

"Oh, Matthew." Heidi pats his back as he pushes his face into the sofa pillow.

He punches the sofa cushion. "I feel like such a baby. Mom and Dad are exhausted. Dad's blood pressure medicine has doubled and Mom has lost ten pounds. I have to be strong. My life has to be on hold for now. Alex is no help; he pops in once or twice a month for a half hour or so."

She nods.

"Denise tells me it's hard to die. She cries whenever we talk about death. Some days she's afraid of dying and other days says it will be a relief, but yesterday she talked about getting better. Then I start crying. But, sometimes we laugh at the good memories we have. It's all hard to deal with."

"The end of life can be a roller coaster. Some people come close to death only to rally for a few days, and then slip back again. It's exhausting for everyone. Take each day as it comes. Ask me for anything you need. I'm here for you."

* * *

Denise soon is too weak to get out of bed.

"She'll likely only live a few more days. Fortunately, she's in no pain," Heidi counsels.

Matthew and his parents are with her the night she dies. The moon is full and its light filters through the windows creating soft shadows on the walls. The quietness should make Matthew feel peaceful and at one with his sister, but it doesn't. Denise is restless.

Matthew runs his fingers across her cheeks. "Don't stay in the world and suffer any more for us. We'll be all right without you." His voice chokes. He's not sure she understands his words, but she becomes calm. Huddled together, the three of them watch life slowly drain from her body.

Once she is gone, Matthew lays his head over his sister's shoulder and weeps. "It's not fair." Tears stream down his face onto her pillow. He runs his fingers over Denise's pale face now hard and cool. Tears in their eyes, his mom and dad stand on the other side of Denise's bed rubbing her arms.

"If only we could breathe life back into her," his mother whispers.

* * *

Later he telephones Heidi. By the time she arrives, Matthew is sitting quietly in his dad's recliner. "I went through the surgery for nothing," he tells the nurse.

"You gave her the gift of time."

Matthew stares out the window as if in a trance. "I feel like a truck has run over me, flattened me out. In the end, I didn't help her at all."

"You gave Denise a longer life. You gave of yourself, did your part. No one can ever take that away from you."

"It wasn't enough. I lost my kidney for nothing. I need to get outta town. I can't stand being in the house with her not here, not hearing her laugh, not getting up at night to cover her when she's cold. I used to sit by her bed and watch just to see that she was still breathing."

Heidi pats his arm. "It's okay to be angry. She left you."

"I know she didn't die on purpose to hurt me." Matthew

155

squeezes his eyes shut.

Heidi leans toward him. "No, but it hurts anyway. There was nothing you could do to keep her alive."

"At first, I prayed to keep her alive. Then, I prayed she would live for just one more day. After that, I prayed her suffering would end."

"She knew you loved her. She told me how much you were there for her. I need to go now, but I'll be back after the funeral. We can talk more then."

"I'll be gone the minute the funeral's over. There's no reason to stay."

"Your mom and dad need you."

He looks at Heidi in despair. "How much more am I supposed to give?"

"Just you being here will help them."

"I can't. It feels like a tomb here. I see Denise everywhere. I hear her voice in the middle of the night, feel her hand in mine. Yet I don't have a sister anymore."

She reaches for his hand. "Maybe your uncle can help."

Matthew nods. "The wheel, the potter's wheel at Uncle Ian's. I'll go there."

* * *

After the funeral, Matthew packs a few things and leaves his parent's house. He heads straight for the potter's wheel in Uncle Ian's studio. The old man is still asleep, and Matthew doesn't wake him. He sits down and picks up the clay and turns it over and over in his hands. When it becomes a smooth ball, he slams it down on the wheel's center. Round and round he spins the wheel working to mold the clay into a flower vase. "I'll put fresh daisies in it every day in her honor," he tells the clay.

Suddenly Denise's presence is near him. His confusion clears and he recognizes that he made the right decision to give his kidney to his sister, that it gave her a chance at life, even though the chance didn't last long.

Matthew wipes his hands on an old towel and fingers the amulet around his neck and thinks about working full-time as a potter. The heck with making money! Kneading the clay gives him peace and an opportunity to make sense of Denise's death. Uncle Ian has the right idea, an introspective life expressing his emotions through art. Matthew smiles as he tries to picture himself as old as Ian. Will he have a beard, too?

Several months later, Matthew quits his job, packs his things, and sublets his townhouse to move to Santa Fe and open an art studio there. He plans to sell his wares, make money, much more than his uncle, get married and have a family.

His business doesn't give him enough income to live comfortably on, so he takes a part-time job teaching pottery at the local community college. Over the years, he finds his life to be more and more like Uncle Ian's, but he's not as eccentric and more social. He becomes a fixture in the town. His former students and the 'locals' stop by his small home studio to talk to him while he turns his potter's wheel. Every time he thinks of Denise, he rolls clay.

There is no wife, no children. His relationships with women don't work out. He finds it too hard to live with anyone for long without becoming sullen and moody.

"You've got loner blood," one girlfriend told him before they broke up.

* * *

The years pass quickly. He makes yearly trips back to Rochester until his mother, father and Uncle Ian die. One day, he is surprised to receive a telephone call from Alex. "I'll be in your area for business. I'd love to stop by for the weekend and help you celebrate your birthday. If I remember right, it's the big "five-oh?"

"Of course, come. I'll be waiting."

Sunday evening, Matthew and Alex sit around Matthew's kitchen table snacking on nachos and a black bean dip.

"Move back to New York," Alex says. "We have more catching up to do. It's just the two of us now with the folks and Uncle Ian gone."

"No, my home's Santa Fe. I've lived here nearly thirty years. You're always welcome," Matthew tells him.

"I know. With my wife working and us needing to baby sit the grandkids, it's hard to travel. I'll be back to visit though," Alex says. "I'll keep in better touch too. It's been good having you around."

"You're a great brother, Matthew. You saved our sister, for a while anyway. I have to admit now, I was glad it wasn't me that had to give up my kidney. I'm sorry I didn't help out more when Denise was dying or visit you the day of the surgery. The day of your operation and the day she died I went to *Smitty's Pub* and got drunk. I'm still afraid of hospitals and operations and, of course, dying."

Matthew nodded. "I was scared out of my mind back then, too. Just did it though. Something got me through, maybe Uncle Ian."

"I didn't help you. I'm sorry."

Matthew leans back in his chair. "It was a bummer. I was angry, especially when she died anyway. And, to be honest, I was mad at you for years. Now I understand. Forget it."

Alex pats his shoulder. "I wasn't there for either of you. But the past is the past. Come on, cheer up. You look beat. It's your birthday. Let's go tie one on."

Matthew looks straight into Alex's eyes and hesitates. "I have bad news, Alex. I can't drink. The doctor says I have end-stage kidney disease too, just like Denise. I've been on dialysis for months."

"God, Matt, what happened?" Alex stares at him in disbelief. "My problem's from diabetes, not related to the transplant, but I need a new kidney. I'm on the waiting list for a cadaver donor."

Matthew sees the blood drain from Alex's face; he thinks his brother might even pass out and curses himself for telling Alex about his kidney failure. Right from the start, he'd promised to keep his health problems to himself.

"I'll do it, little brother, get re-tested." Alex gulps. "It's the right thing for me to do. If you did it, so can I. A family member is best. I remember that from Dr. Lyon."

"There's laparoscopic surgery now. It's easier."

"There are better medicines, too. I probably won't be a perfect match, but the new immunosuppressant medications should prevent rejection."

Matthew smiles gently at his older brother. His left hand fingers the Uncle Ian's clay amulet around his neck. With his right hand, he picks up a ball of clay from a nearby table and throws it at his brother. "Thanks for coming, Alex."

Alex catches the clay ball one-handed and throws it back. "Happy Birthday, Matt."

Matthew laughs as he grabs the clay from the air and lays it back on the table. "You'll need a wheel before this is over." Then, he engulfs Alex in a long bear hug.

BIOGRAPHY

Lois Gerber, RN believes in the spirit of community health nursing—its focus on wellness, relationships, families, and communities. Her BSN, MPH in Nursing, and Specialist in Aging certificate opened many professional doors. She's worked in home health agencies, public health departments, and an Area Agency on Aging. She's taught nursing students on the university level and has counseled families dealing with elder care issues. For forty some years, Lois has helped people of all ages, various religions and ethnicities, and different socio-economic levels. These stories reflect her experiences.